D1266463

EMOTIONALLY FOCUSED COUPLE THERAPY WITH TRAUMA SURVIVORS

The Guilford Family Therapy Series

Michael P. Nichols, *Series Editor*

Emotionally Focused Couple Therapy with Trauma Survivors

Strengthening Attachment Bonds

SUSAN M. JOHNSON

THE GUILFORD PRESS
New York   London

© 2002 Susan M. Johnson
Published by The Guilford Press
A Division of Guilford Publications, Inc.
72 Spring Street, New York, NY 10012
www.guilford.com

Printed in the United States of America

This book is printed on acid-free paper.

Last digit is print number: 9   8   7   6   5   4   3   2

Library of Congress Cataloging-in-Publication Data

Johnson, Susan M.
    Emotionally focused couple therapy with trauma survivors :
strengthening attachment bonds / Susan M. Johnson.
        p. cm. — (The Guilford family therapy series)
    Includes bibliographical references and index.
    ISBN 1-57230-735-8 (hard)
        1. Marital psychotherapy. 2. Attachment behavior. 3. Psychic
trauma—Patients—Family relationships. I. Title. II. Series.

    RC488.5 .J589 2002
    616.89'156—dc21   2001056916

To all the couples who, as John Bowlby put it many years ago, have worked so hard to educate me—especially to those who, having seen the worst in their fellow human beings, still hope and struggle to trust and connect.

About the Author

Susan M. Johnson has a doctorate in counseling psychology and is a registered psychologist in the city of Ottawa, Canada. She is one of the originators and the main proponent of emotionally focused couple therapy. This approach, which is also used with families, integrates experiential and systemic perspectives and has been extensively empirically validated. Dr. Johnson is Professor of Psychology at the University of Ottawa and Director of the Ottawa Couple and Family Institute. She is also Research Professor in the Marital and Family Therapy Program at Alliant International University in San Diego, California. In 2000, she received the American Association for Marriage and Family Therapy Outstanding Contribution to the Field Award. She is a well-known international presenter on couple therapy, adult attachment, emotion in psychotherapy, and working with traumatized couples. (Note: For more information on emotionally focused couple therapy on the Internet, go to www.eft.ca.)

Preface

*T*he field of couple therapy is entering a new era. No beginning couple therapist now has to walk into his or her first session without a sense of what the significant landmarks are in the vast and confusing landscape of relationship distress. Research tells us, for example, that the inability to offer comfort or stay emotionally engaged is at least as important as, if not more important than, how many times a couple fights or whether they resolve their arguments. The beginning couple therapist now also has a theory of love and relatedness to draw on in the form of attachment theory. It can be argued that before this theory was applied to adult relationships, the therapist had very sparse resources in terms of a theory of adult love to guide goal setting and intervention. Attachment theory offers the therapist a map of the territory of adult love relationships. We also have models of intervention that have been specified and tested.

This is a very different field from the one I entered 20 years ago. As it becomes clear that the quality of our attachment relationships has an enormous impact on our everyday lives, our physical and mental health, and how we see ourselves, it makes sense that couple interventions are beginning to address issues that used to be the exclusive territory of the individual therapist—issues such as depression and, as presented in this text, disorders of posttraumatic stress.

The ultimate message of systems theory is that an individual's adjustment problems are best seen and understood in the context of that individual's interactions with others, especially in the context of his or her patterns of interaction with family and loved ones. This book is completely consistent with this systemic tradition and focuses on the power of close relationships not only to ignite or maintain such adjustment problems, but also to heal them. John Bowlby, the father of attachment theory, believed that the development of love was the crowning achievement of human evolution. It is also, if expressed and accepted, the logical antidote to the helplessness and sense of isolation and betrayal that are the essence of so many traumatic experiences.

However, if you had asked me a few years ago whether couple therapy could really make a difference to the partners in a distressed relationship in which one partner was struggling with posttraumatic stress disorder, particularly when this disorder was complex and chronic, I probably would have expressed doubt. I would have felt daunted by the scale and complexity of the task. The traumatized couples with whom my colleagues and I worked in the marital and family clinic of the Ottawa Civic Hospital changed my mind. Trauma survivors showed me that they were more than willing, even if they had been terribly wounded by significant others, to fight their fears and to struggle to create a new kind of connection with their present partners. These partners also showed me that they were capable of more generous and compassionate understanding and care than I had imagined possible. Moreover, a new sense of felt security in this couple relationship seemed to open a direct route to individual healing for the survivor.

At the same time my client couples were educating me, the trauma literature began to focus ever more on the power of emotional bonds to significant others to soothe anxiety and create resilience. But this focus on the role of such bonds did not seem to extend to the area of clinical intervention, except perhaps in the context of the therapeutic relationship between an individual therapist and his or her client. This book integrates the recent work on adult attachment, the recent links between attachment and healing delineated in the trauma literature, our evolving understanding of the nature of traumatic stress, and clinical interventions in couple therapy.

After an introductory chapter, the first half of the book offers a brief review of the nature of trauma, the nature of attachment, and the relevance of an attachment perspective for trauma survivors and their partners. Chapter 4 addresses assessment issues with traumatized couples. Chapter 5 outlines interventions across different stages of treatment with couples facing trauma. These stages are, first, the creation of stability and de-escalation of trauma symptoms and relationship distress; second, the restructuring of interactions so as to create the secure bonding that fosters individual and relationship healing; and, finally, the integration of these changes into the life of the couple and each partner's engagement with the effects of trauma. (Note: The general web site for emotionally focused couple therapy is www.eft.ca.)

The second half of the book consists largely of clinical case studies of couple therapy with couples facing particular traumas. These cases include couples who are fighting for their relationships while dealing with the aftermath of trauma arising from combat, the trauma of mental illness and physical illness, and violence and sexual abuse in previous relationships. There is also a chapter on what my colleagues and I call attachment injuries or relationship traumas. These injuries involve incidents in which a partner's lack of responsiveness at a time of extreme need was in itself traumatic and defined an attachment relationship as unsafe, so that it could not provide a haven in times of stress. These relationship traumas also create impasses in the creation of more secure bonds in couple therapy. The final chapter considers the role of the therapist and the challenge and promise of working with couples facing trauma.

I would like to thank my colleagues who worked on my team at the Civic Hospital and at the Ottawa Couple and Family Institute for their support, enthusiasm, and creativity. I would also like to thank my students at the University of Ottawa, Department of Psychology, for constantly asking questions and bringing me clinical dilemmas, then helping me find the answers to those dilemmas. Thanks also to the editors at The Guilford Press, Jim Nageotte and Mike Nichols, for their support. I am particularly grateful to my friend and colleague Lyn Williams Keeler, MA, who was the primary author of Chapter 9 of this book and was the therapist in the case. Lyn specializes in the treatment of combat posttraumatic stress disorder and has a wealth of experience in working with veterans. She presents regularly at the conferences of the International Society for Traumatic Stress Studies. I must also say that without the loving support and constant help and encouragement of my husband, John Palmer Douglas, writing this book would not have been possible. Most of all, however, this book is written as a tribute to my clients, who constantly humble and amaze me with their courage and strength and who constantly teach me, not just about how we shape our most important relationships, but about what it means to be human. Throughout the book I refer to the helplessness and terror that survivors of trauma face every day as "the dragon"—an archetypal image of humankind's deepest fears and a reminder that we all have potential to be heroes and to face those fears.

Contents

Part I

Trauma in Context: Healing in Attachment Relationships

Chapter 1

Healing Connections: Expanding the Role of Couple Therapy

*I*n old Celtic stories, where life is dark and full of danger, poets and seers teach people how to face the darkness. They teach that life is about standing in a narrow passage, in the dark, with your back against the wall, facing a dragon. There is no escape. The only question, in these old stories, is how well you fight. This is a somber vision, but also one that celebrates the courage that the darkness calls forth.

To those of us who see the power of intimate bonds, in couples and in families, there is a second question: the question of whether you fight alone.

If another stands beside you when you face overwhelming terror and helplessness—whether you name this terror and helplessness a "dragon" or call it by some other name, such as traumatic stress—then everything is different. Shadows are not so terrifying. The struggle can be shared, and sometimes the fight can even be a thing of joy as, together, you defy the dragon. We all know it is better not to be alone in the dark and that connection with others makes us stronger.

This knowledge is the basis of the entire enterprise called psychotherapy. Every therapist knows that when we are wounded, connection with another helps us heal. The one thread that has united therapists across models and paradigms is a recognition that the relationship with a therapist is a new context that can create new, healing experiences for clients. Research on the effects of psychotherapy has echoed this recognition. More essential than the use of technical skill is "being skillfully" with our clients. If a therapist is a skilled weaver of new realities, the therapeutic relationship is the frame on which such realities are woven and become tangible.

Couple and family therapists attempt to create new, more positive connections, not only between the therapist and individual clients, but between family members. We have been intent on improving couple relationships and helping families to step out of negative ways of relating. We have tried to help people resolve conflicts, communicate more effectively, and create greater intimacy. And, if we consider couple therapy, the subject of this book, we seem to have made headway in helping couples improve distressed relationships. There are now a number of empirically validated couple therapies, and in the last decade this field has made strides in identifying common relationship problems and ways to alleviate those problems (Johnson & Lebow, 2000). Recently, couple therapy has also been used to address "individual" problems such as depression and anxiety disorders, agoraphobia, addictions, and eating disorders (Baucom, Shoham, Mueser, Daiuto, & Stickle, 1998). It may be used as a main intervention or as an adjunct to more individually focused interventions. For example, Barlow and colleagues (Barlow, O'Brien, & Last, 1984; Cerny, Barlow, Craske, & Himadi, 1987) found that when spouses were included in treatment for anxiety, success rates jumped from 46 to 82%. The growing trend to use couple interventions to address common problems of individuals is a recognition of the importance of our closest relationships in our lives. These relationships can maintain and exacerbate personal problems; they can also be active sources of healing.

This book reflects and extends this trend in the evolution of the field of couple therapy. It concerns the use of couple therapy, not only to alleviate relationship distress and to help individuals address problems of mental and physical health, but also to help couples construct relationships that enable partners to face the traumas inflicted by life and to walk away from them whole.

Trauma involves exposure to a stressor that evokes intense fear, helplessness, and horror. This experience irrevocably shapes the way a survivor defines the world and his or her self. Trauma may involve echoes from the past, such as childhood sexual abuse (CSA). This form of trauma, often inflicted by those we need most, has a powerful effect on how people construct their lives and their relationships. In fact, the effects of CSA are so patent as to be given special recognition and are now referred to as complex posttraumatic stress disorder. Trauma may also involve present trials, such as physical or mental illness, the traumatic loss of a loved one, and the occupational traumas that soldiers and police officers face daily. These traumas are not inflicted by loved ones, but the aftereffects are played out in technicolor in the victim's close relationships, often with disastrous results. The thesis of this book is that couple therapy has a vital role to play in addressing the interpersonal effects of trauma and helping partners to turn their relationship into a safe haven, a haven that actively promotes facing the dragon well and healing from the aftereffects of his fire.

This broader view of the role of couple therapy fits with the heightened awareness of the last decade that couple interventions can be actively used to promote health and resilience in individual partners. New approaches to couple therapy have tended to depathologize relationship problems and emphasize the resources partners may have to offer each other. For example, emotionally focused and narrative therapies both take such a stance (Freedman & Combs, 1996; Johnson, 1996). Our closest relationships can provide the ideal context in which we can heal and grow (Hendrix, 1988; Johnson, 1986; Walsh, 1996). Couple and family therapists are now focusing not just on resolving relationship problems, but on specific ways in which better relationships can promote positive coping and individual growth. In this context, it makes sense that improving an individual's closest relationships can be a crucial element in addressing multidimensional problems that involve the whole personality, such as posttraumatic stress disorder (PTSD).

This expanded view of the potential role of couple therapy is supported by a convergence of philosophical perspectives that focus on changing the relationship context in which an individual problem is enacted. The feminist movement offers one such perspective. Feminists and other writers are emphasizing that the self is relational, that we define ourselves in relation to others (Jordan, Kaplan, Miller, Stiver, & Surrey, 1991) and that man is a mirror for man. This argument echoes Sullivan (1953), who talked many years ago about how personality is the way we engage with others and create social relationships. Social psychologists, who study attachment between intimates, view a person's style of engagement with others as intimately connected to his or her model of self and how emotion and information are processed in everyday life (Bartholomew & Horowitz, 1991). Postmodern social constructionists also emphasize how the sense of self is continually created in interaction with others (Anderson, 1997). All these theorists stress that identity is not so much an achievement of the mind, but a reflection of key relationships and a drama requiring a supporting cast (Gergen, 1994). These perspectives add momentum to the use of couple therapy to address problems that until recently were considered the exclusive domain of long-term individual therapy.

Advances in the couple therapy field also make this modality more applicable to serious individual problems. It is significant that couple therapists are focusing not just on behaviors in interactions but also on emotions in the change process. This focus helps the couple therapist to specifically address an individual partner's emotional problems, particularly traumatic stress disorders, in which emotional regulation and integration are of such central importance. Recent advances in the literature on the use of emotion in clinical practice point out that emotion bridges self and system, the intrapsychic and interpersonal worlds (Greenberg, Rice, & Elliott, 1993; Kennedy-Moore & Watson, 1999; Plutchik, 2000). Emotion orients us to the salience of events, colors the meaning of these events, and primes us for action. It also structures communications with others and evokes particular responses from them. Thus, sadness can speak to me of my loss and bring that loss into focus. It moves me to weep and seek comfort. Its expression also conveys to my partner that I need soothing and draws him or her closer (Johnson & Greenberg, 1994). Couple therapists who work with emotional realities and emotional communication are in a unique position to impact clients' inner and relational worlds. It is logical that as an intimate relationship improves, the individual partner's sense of self and general resources for dealing with life's challenges also improve. It is perhaps not so easy to recognize that couple therapy may provide a unique arena for specific and crucial changes in individual functioning. When a survivor is able, in spite of terror and shame, to turn to his or her partner and ask to be held and comforted during a flashback, rather than to dissociate or harm him- or herself, not only are the negative symptoms of PTSD modified, but a new world of trust and a new sense of self open for that survivor.

This book suggests that for many clients, particularly those struggling with the aftermath of a trauma characterized by "violations of human connection" (Herman, 1992), there is a potentially more powerful corrective relationship than the relationship with a therapist. This is the relationship with the person's life partner. This relationship is often overlooked or discounted by health professionals as an active source of healing. It is addressed, if at all, only when distress between partners clearly and irrevocably undermines the effectiveness of one partner's individual therapy. This book focuses particularly on the aftereffects of different kinds of trauma and takes the position that if a person's connection with significant others is not part of the coping and healing process, then, inevitably, it becomes part of the problem and even a source of retraumatization. As healers, we may sometimes forget the brilliance of ordinary people in healing themselves and the people they love. My client couples have taught me that, in general, we underestimate the ability of a husband to comfort his wife when a traumatic flashback wakes her in the middle of the night. We tend to forget the powerful, positive impact of such events on a survivor. As therapists, we may have focused too much on the individual and underutilized the power of a client's attachment to a significant other as a natural and potent antidote to helplessness and loss. Perhaps the field of couple therapy is now ready to take up the challenge, not only of healing relationships, but of helping couples create relationships that heal the traumatic wounds that life inflicts on so many of us.

Why is this the time for the field of couple therapy to address such a challenge ?

First, couple therapy as a modality has evolved to the point where we have a clear sense of the nature of distress in close relationships, as well as well delineated and tested interventions such as emotionally focused couple therapy. We can have increased confidence in our ability to help couples, even very distressed couples who are dealing with symptoms such as depression and PTSD, to change their relationships for the better.

Second, there is accumulating evidence of the effect of close relationships on physical and mental health and the ability to cope with stress. Positive close relationships have been linked to immune system competence, to resilience in combat situations, and to the ability to cope with chronic stress and illness (Kiecolt-Glasser et al., 1993). Conversely, there is increasing recognition of the links between relationship distress and emotional problems, particularly depression and posttraumatic stress disorder (Whisman, 1999). As "social capital"—that is, our sense of community—diminishes and the anxiety and stress involved in everyday life increase (Twenge, 2000), it may be that we need ever more support from our partners and have fewer other resources when these relationships become distressed.

Third, a theory of adult love relationships has been elaborated that allows us to clearly conceptualize and explain the link between secure relationships with others and the development of personal resilience. We now have a theory that explains how being connected with others enables us to overcome fears and maintain resilience. Attachment theory (Bowlby, 1969) specifies that secure bonds foster our ability to cope with hurt and danger, whereas isolation and alienation from others render us vulnerable.

Fourth, and perhaps most significant, in the last decade the enormous impact of traumatic experience, particularly physical and sexual abuse, on people's emotional and physical health has been recognized. In particular, there has been greater recognition of the "violation of human connection" (Herman, 1992) that occurs when trauma is inflicted by those we depend on and are closest to. This kind of experience is *not* rare or unusual. Herman (1981) suggests that up to one-third of all women have had some form of sexual experience with a male relative while growing up. In response to this awareness, a plethora of new interventions have evolved, most of them directed at the survivor as an individual (Foa & Rothbaum, 1998). In addition, it has been acknowledged that these interventions must be efficient and, where possible, brief.

Finally, we now better understand traumatic experience in terms of both its multidimensional nature and its far-reaching effects, and thus we see the need to intervene on a number of levels, including a victim's interpersonal context. There is a growing recognition that although re-experiencing symptoms are being successfully treated with interventions such as exposure-based therapies (Foa, Hearst-Ikeda, & Perry, 1995), the interpersonal symptoms of trauma, such as numbing and detachment, are difficult to treat via the traditional individually focused interventions. Symptoms such as numbing and hyperawareness may be best addressed by the comfort and reassurance offered by a significant other.

The multidimensional nature of the aftereffects of trauma implies that to effectively treat trauma, we need to use different interventions to hit different targets. However, treatment has mostly focused on the inner experience of the individual survivor, with the additional use of structured group experiences. Until quite recently, couple therapy has not been employed systematically to address the effects of trauma, even though distressed relationships are such a central feature of posttraumatic stress.

Perhaps because more of the work in this field has focused on the female survivor of trauma (except in combat stress disorders), as a colleague has suggested, men have been seen as the enemy, not part of the healing. But this perspective ignores the many female survivors with long-term partners who are spending a great part of their lives struggling to connect to these partners, in spite of their traumatic experiences. When we consider survivors who have coped with childhood trauma successfully, we see that a positive relationship with an adult partner is often a key factor in their success. Women who have been abused as children and are able to be good parents for their own children, for example, are often those who have managed to create a positive relationship with a spouse, in spite of the lack of maps or models. At first, as couple therapists, my colleagues and I simply saw that helping couples improve their relationship often took longer if one partner had a trauma history. It took time for couples to teach us that when partners successfully fight the dragon of trauma together, not only is the dragon more likely to be put in its place, but the fight builds a powerful bond between the partners. Our couples helped us to see that a partner who understands the nature of the terror that takes over his or her spouse is often capable of more empathy and responsiveness than we or the survivor had ever imagined possible. Not only that, a spouse or lover is there in the middle of the night when the dragon comes, whereas the therapist, no matter how expert and empathic, is miles away. The fact that if partners are not part of the solution, they are, almost inevitably, part of the problem, is also a cogent argument for couple interventions. If a partner does not understand and is unable to respond to the survivor's pain, however expressed, that partner most often confirms the survivor's worst fears and exacerbates his or her difficulties. This argument is not meant to imply that individual therapy is less than essential in the majority of cases. Rather, it posits that couple interventions can make a crucial, and to date almost unrecognized, contribution in the treatment of traumatic stress.

Perhaps we have not generally used couple therapy to address post-traumatic stress because we have not been sufficiently clear about the impact of trauma on close relationships to know what to target in therapy. We were unclear about where and how to intervene and the best ways to help restore and empower such relationships. If, in the past, we have been unsure about how to promote couple relationships as positive sources of healing for individual wounds, we may now be at the point where we can realistically think of intervening to create specific

changes in individual functioning, as well as to the nature of relationships.

This book is intended as a guide for the therapist working with
couples who are struggling with the impact of trauma on their relationships, seeking to create secure bonds that promote healing for the survivor. More generally, this text will have relevance for therapists in helping couples deal with other "individual" disorders, such as depression
and eating disorders. If the marital relationship is seen as a key factor in
the trauma recovery environment, and if we acknowledge that marital
distress tends to evoke and maintain trauma symptoms, we must pay
attention to the quality of survivors' primary relationships. Van der
Kolk and his colleagues (van der Kolk, Perry, & Herman, 1991) state
that it is the ability to derive comfort from another human being that
ultimately determines the aftermath of trauma, not the history of the
trauma itself. For traumatized couples, *the therapist's goal must be not
just to lessen the distress in a survivor's relationship, but to create the
secure attachment that promotes active and optimal adaptation to a
world that contains danger and terror, but is not necessarily defined by
it.*

Trauma intensifies the need for protective attachments and often,
simultaneously, destroys the ability to trust that is the basis of such attachments. The couple therapist is therefore likely to see a disproportionate number of trauma survivors in his or her practice. Trauma survivors are more likely to experience distress in their close relationships
and to have fewer resources to deal with this distress. Much of their energy is consumed in facing a world infused with danger and uncertainty.
They are more likely to get stuck in the deadly cycles of pursue–
withdraw and criticize–defend that consume relationships and make
separation so likely (Gottman, 1994). It makes ultimate sense that after
experiencing a traumatic disruption or betrayal of human connection,
they have difficulty with trust and closeness and are generally reluctant
to risk that kind of hurt again. However, without this human connection, they cannot truly heal.

From my experience in our hospital clinic, survivors and their partners tend to be caught in a relentless spiral in which relationship distress
primes and exacerbates trauma symptoms, and trauma symptoms
prime and exacerbate relationship distress. This spiral takes on a life of
its own, becomes self-reinforcing, and is often the reason that individual
therapists send their clients to a couple therapist. The survivor's partner

is, at one moment, a potential source of safety and healing, and at the next moment, a source of danger and fear.

THE SCOPE OF THIS TEXT

This text offers a general approach to therapy with traumatized couples, for whom affect regulation and safe emotional engagement are key issues. It can hopefully be useful for all couple therapists, regardless of their theoretical orientation. This is an attempt to go beyond the specific model of therapy with which I am most familiar, emotionally focused couple therapy (EFT; Greenberg & Johnson, 1988; Johnson, 1996). Interventions based on other constructionist therapies, such as narrative therapy, and more dynamic approaches are discussed when they seem to have something to offer the therapist dealing with trauma survivors. Constructivist therapies, such as EFT, focus on human beings as active agents who individually and collectively construct the meaning of their experiential world (Neimeyer, 1993). Such therapies tend to focus on the process of meaning creation, on the self in relation to others, and on the manner in which individuals organize themselves and their experiences to protect their internal coherence and integrity.

This text, however, takes a particular theoretical perspective on adult love, an attachment perspective. Currently, this perspective is supported by the most extensive research base of any theory of adult love and offers couple therapists of all persuasions a general map of close relationships. It is also particularly pertinent to trauma survivors and their relationships. Attachment theory stresses that emotional ties with others, wired in by evolution, offer all of us a safe haven in times of need and a secure base from which to explore and learn to survive in a dangerous world. A secure connection with others is most pertinent in the face of danger and loss. The lack of such connection not only leaves us unprotected but can, in itself, be aversive and even traumatic. Confinement in solitary isolation, often called cruel and unusual punishment in our penal systems, is used as a general means of torture to deliberately induce helplessness and terror, that is, to induce traumatic stress.

This text also examines negative events that violate the assumptions of attachment relationships, just as trauma tends to violate the individual's assumptions about a safe and controllable world. Conceptualizing these injuries as relationship traumas has helped my colleagues and me to grasp, understand, and design interventions to address such injuries. If unresolved, these injuries block the growth of trust and openness in couples' relationships and undermine the effectiveness of couple therapy (Johnson, Makinen, & Millikin, 2001).

We begin with some brief snapshots of the kinds of issues these couples bring to therapy.

SOME SNAPSHOTS: COUPLES FACING TRAUMA

Relational cues to the presence of the dragon

WIFE: Don't just come up behind me and grab me—like you did last night. I hate it.

HUSBAND: What do you mean? I don't know how to be with you. I can't even give you a hug without you going off the deep end.

WIFE: Just don't do it. It's aggressive. It's just like I'm back home with my brothers—always touching me, touching me. (*Shudders and starts to cry.*)

HUSBAND: (*deep sigh*) Fine, fine. I will just stay away from you then.

Dealing with re-experiencing problems

WIFE: When you have these, these nightmares, why don't you tell me, wake me up?

HUSBAND: Oh yeah, right. Then you could tell your friends—"He lost it again last night, some kind of cop he is. One shoot-out and he turns into some kind of pathetic crybaby who's afraid of the dark." Just leave me alone.

Numbing and dissociation

HUSBAND: I don't feel anything right now. When she cries like this, I just hear that I have screwed up again. Like I did in the fire that night. It's like I'm a long way off. I'm hardly even here.

WIFE: That's right—you are never with me when I need you. What's the point?

Avoidance

WIFE: I can't handle. it. I don't mind a cuddle, in fact, it helps sometimes. But I can't handle it when I see that look in his eye. He wants sex. So I go on the computer for a few hours.

HUSBAND: When we were first together, you wanted sex all the time. Now I can't even touch you. Why am I here? You don't want me at all.

Hypervigilance

WIFE: I'm on eggshells all the time. Everything has to be perfect, in place, predictable. And if it isn't, well, all hell breaks loose and I am the enemy.

HUSBAND: I know, I know. But if you would just keep everything. . . . All right, I know, I am so thin-skinned, I'm bleeding to death here.

Irritability

HUSBAND: You're angry all the time, with me, with the kids. You got assaulted, okay, but you know, we aren't the ones who assaulted you. But we are the ones that get to pay for it and we've paid for it for a long time now. When is it going to stop ?

WIFE: (*in a dull, listless voice*) It's never stopped—never going to stop—that's the point.

From the preceding examples, it is easy to get a sense of how the aftermath of trauma interferes with emotional engagement in a relationship and how this lack of safe engagement then plays a part in maintaining traumatic stress. The couple therapist has the perspective and the expertise to help such couples create new kinds of interactions whereby the echoes of trauma can be contained and the wounds associated with it can be healed.

Chapter 2

Trauma and Its Aftermath

*T*rauma is defined in the dictionary as a wound. More specifically, trauma occurs when a person is confronted with a threat to the physical integrity of self or another, a threat that overwhelms coping resources and evokes subjective responses of intense terror, helplessness, and horror. Trauma nearly always involves a sense of loss. It is a moment when we can see the world shift and turn, understanding that neither we nor the world will ever be the same. Once we have been so wounded, we are faced with our own vulnerability in an irrevocable and palpable way.

This book looks at trauma as classically defined—for example, trauma arising from war and rape. It also considers childhood sexual abuse, recognized as a special kind of trauma in which inescapable shock often disrupts developmental processes and leads to what has been referred to as *complex* posttraumatic stress disorders (Chu, 1998; Herman, 1992). This is a form of trauma in which close relationships themselves become contaminated with the terror of past traumas and so cannot act as a context for healing. Almost everyone would agree that trauma has occurred in these situations—war, rape, childhood abuse—and we can expect that a certain number of victims will suffer from partial or full-blown PTSD and a variety of other symptoms, particularly depression.

The book also discusses traumatic situations in which people find themselves facing mental and physical illness, illnesses that change their existential reality and their relationships. We do not usually speak of these experiences in the same breath with the wounds of war and rape, even if they can sometimes elicit the same intense fear and helplessness. However, when such illnesses arise, many couples seek out a couple therapist to assist them in limiting the impact of traumatic stress on their relationship and helping each other through these crises.

The book goes on to examine what we call attachment injuries (Johnson & Whiffen, 1999; Johnson et al., 2001). These are wounds arising from abandonment by a present attachment figure in a situation of urgent need. These injuries become touchstones that define a relationship as insecure and undependable and leave individual partners facing the trauma of separateness and isolation. For example, a woman tells her spouse that she has just discovered she has breast cancer. Her spouse does not respond to her disclosure. In fact, he immediately leaves the room and later announces he has to leave for a week on a business trip. When we face the dragon alone, the aloneness itself is traumatizing. Abandonment by an attachment figure in the face of threat is not simply a very unpleasant experience. It has an evolutionary significance. Relevant research shows that isolation is just as dangerous as smoking, high blood pressure, and cholesterol (House, Landis, & Umberson, 1988). It removes our main buffer against disorganizing stress and helplessness, namely, our connection with each other.

Recent trauma research suggests that we are a resilient species. Many of us find ways to recover from traumatic experience, or at least to bear our scars in a way that allows us to live relatively fulfilling lives. Even so, the debilitating symptoms of posttraumatic stress are not rare, particularly in people who seek out a therapist. Some researchers have reported that as many as 13% of women in the United States are victims of a forcible rape in their lifetime, most of which will never be reported (Resnick, Kilpatrick, Dansky, Saunders, & Best, 1993). Up to 46% of these women will suffer the symptoms of PTSD, and the prevalence of rates of PTSD among men who are raped are even higher. A study of female rape and crime victims also found that 16.5% of the victims met the criteria for PTSD some 15 years after the assault (Keesler, Sonnega, Bromet, Hughes, & Nelson, 1995; Kilpatrick, Saunders, Veranen, Best, & Van, 1987). If we simply consider CSA, it is estimated that as many as 20% of female children are sexually abused in their own families by a family member and approximately 5% report father–daughter incest (Badgely et al., 1984; Finkelhor, 1984; Russell, 1984). In a large national sample in the United States, 12.3% of women reported having PTSD at some point in their lifetimes, and 4.6% were experiencing PTSD at the time of the study (Resnick et al., 1993). According to a 1990 study (Breslau, Davis, Andreski, & Peterson, 1991) more than 9% of people in an urban suburb were suffering from PTSD. This is the same rate of prevalence as generally found for major depression. As Foa and Rothbaum (1998) point out, PTSD poses a serious health problem in North America, especially for women.

It is also becoming clear that a large proportion of outpatients displaying a wide range of symptoms are incest survivors. When these individuals' symptoms are not seen in the context of the trauma they have endured, they tend to be labeled by the helping professions as personality disorders, particularly as borderline personality disorder. In our couple and family therapy clinic, we would often see victims of incest with full and partial PTSD and the comorbid symptoms of severe depression, suicidal behavior, eating disorders and anxiety disorders. Most often these clients are referred because individual or group therapy for their individual symptoms has reached an impasse. Clients often state that distress in their primary relationship preoccupies and paralyzes them, exacerbating their PTSD symptoms and impeding their progress in other therapy modalities. Charlene, a CSA survivor whose relationship is described in Chapter 6, said, "When I realized how distant we'd become, everything went over the top. All the feelings of being contaminated and despicable flooded me. The only way out was less of me. So I stopped eating and stopped feeling. I couldn't really respond to the therapists in the eating disorders clinic. As soon as I got home, this would all take over again."

THE NATURE OF POSTTRAUMATIC STRESS DISORDER

PTSD first became recognized as a formal diagnosis by the American Psychiatric Association in 1980. The symptoms of what we now refer to as PTSD had been outlined earlier by pioneers such as Charcot, Janet, Breuer, and Freud, particularly in relation to hysteria in women, and subsequently by therapists such as Kardiner (1941) who studied mental breakdown in those who fought in the world wars. It is interesting for our purposes to note that Kardiner and Spiegel (1947) state that the strongest protection against overwhelming terror in war seemed to be the degree of relatedness, the bond, between fighting men. In the mid-1970s the veterans of Vietnam educated us about the nature of trauma to the point where the effects of trauma were finally formally recognized by health professionals. Since that time there has been an increasing focus on what Herman (1992) calls the "combat neurosis of the sex war," that is, the effects of childhood sexual abuse on the lives of women. Rape has been identified as the archetypal image of inescapable shock, and there is also increasing recognition that men too can be victims. Contributors such as Foa and her colleagues (Foa, Hearst-Ikeda, & Perry, 1995; Foa & Riggs, 1993) have outlined the wide-ranging effects of sexual violence on women and outlined and tested behavioral therapeutic interventions to help individuals deal with the intrusive symptoms of trauma.

There is general agreement that traumatic experience, where neither resistance nor escape is possible, overwhelms ordinary human regulatory processes and is fundamentally disorganizing. Inner and outer worlds are rendered chaotic and unpredictable. Janet (1909), one of the first to identify posttraumatic stress, wrote of the "dissolving" effects of the strong emotions aroused by trauma, and modern authors stress that the primary effect of trauma is a chronic inability to regulate one's emotional life. Survivors also speak of the debilitating sense that what they most trusted, their own minds, seem to have turned against them.

We, as mental health professionals, are still struggling to grasp and identify the essential features of traumatic stress responses. There is some debate about how posttraumatic stress responses should be generally categorized. Specifically, should PTSD be viewed as primarily a disorder of dissociation or, as it is now categorized in the fourth edition of the *Diagnostic and Statistical Manual of Mental Disorders* (DSM-IV; American Psychiatric Association, 1994), as a disorder of anxiety? Most clinicians, however, view a traumatic stress response as a process characterized by terror and helplessness, which then often narrows and constricts the focus of a person's life and prevents new learning. Trauma survivors' engagement with their own experiences and with the world become dominated by issues of safety and survival, and thus by habitual fight, flight, and freeze responses that can become self-perpetuating and prevent engagement in new and potentially healing experiences. The primary symptoms of PTSD noted in DSM-IV are as follows:

1. *Intrusive re-experiencing.* Re-experiencing episodes often take the form of dreams or intrusive thoughts and powerful emotional reactions to internal or external cues linked to a trauma. These cues may be events that most of us would find rewarding, such as being held by our partner, but can suddenly become aversive for the survivors of trauma.

This symptom also involves being "there rather than here," as in flash-back experiences. This intrusive re-experiencing undermines the survi-vor's sense of control and reinforces the belief that terror and helpless-ness, the dragon of trauma, can come for him or her at any time. It also undermines connections with others, who are often experienced as peripheral at such times. Survivors are caught and absorbed in the re-experiencing and are seen by their partners as absent and disengaged.

2. *Numbing and avoidance.* The avoidance of trauma triggers may seem to be a natural response to overwhelming trauma. Unfortunately for many survivors, avoidance of trauma cues means being unable to engage in the daily activities that make life worthwhile. Sarah could not take a shower. Her ex-husband used to attack her savagely in the shower. Marie, who, as a child, was continually raped by her older brothers, has to systematically numb herself to engage in any kind of sexual activity, even though she loves her husband. Although avoidance and numbing are often linked, there is evidence that numbing, or the shutting down of the affective system, is, in fact, separate from avoid-ance and is a reaction to the other symptoms of traumatic stress (Foa & Rothbaum, 1998). Horowitz (1986) suggests that a cycle of intrusive symptoms, which he views as attempts to complete and integrate the trauma, followed by numbing and dissociation to cope with such symp-toms, is the essence of posttraumatic stress. Numbing has also been linked to the physical depletion that results from hyperarousal (Litz et al., 1997). Attempts at suppressing emotional experience, such as numbing, are often ineffective, leading to greater physiological arousal and disturbance (Gross & Levenson, 1993). This symptom, which in-volves restricted affect and detachment from others, appears to be more difficult to treat than other symptoms and predicts distress in a survi-vor's relationships (Riggs, Byrne, Weathers, & Litz, 1998). It is also as-sociated with major depression.

3. *Hyperarousal symptoms.* Sleep disturbances, profound hyper-vigilance and exaggerated startle responses, poor concentration and ir-ritability are often part of PTSD. In couple therapy with trauma survi-vors the modulation of anger and irritability is often a central issue. One survivor described this experience in terms of having no skin, so that every stimulus, every touch from her partner, was experienced as a potential threat and evoked agitation in her. As Waites (1993) suc-cinctly puts it, for survivors the "internal warning system, originally a normal survival mechanism, has gone awry and is now a problem rather than a solution" (p. 22).

This list of symptoms, which reflects mostly the experience of male war veterans, does not capture the complex problems of many survivors, particularly those who were abused as children or who have suffered multiple traumas. For a formal diagnosis of PTSD, one intrusive, three avoidance /numbing, and two hyperarousal symptoms are necessary. However, many of the problems arising from trauma are relatively unrecognized in this formulation. It is also rare for PTSD to appear alone. Trauma itself, and the secondary difficulties that arise in coping with trauma symptoms, make the occurrence of additional problems such as major depression extremely likely.

Feminist conceptualizations of trauma are critical of the narrowness of the range of experiences considered traumatic on the basis of DSM criteria (Root, 1992; Waites, 1993). They point to evidence that traumatic events are not "uncommon," as suggested in the DSM. In the lives of many women and children, they are more like everyday occurrences. Data from DSM field trials also suggest that a strict interpretation of criterion A, that trauma results from uncommon experience, is inappropriate. In these trials it was clear that a high percentage of subjects who had experienced relatively low-magnitude stressor events suffer from significant PTSD symptomatology (Litz & Weathers, 1994). Several authors have suggested changing DSM's coverage of PTSD by including a focus on subjective judgments about what constitutes a traumatic event and stressing perceived helplessness and/or lack of control as well as the severity of the experience.

Feminist authors also focus on the need for greater recognition of the individual's perspective on what is traumatic and emphasize the complex effects of traumas that occur in childhood (Zlotnick et al., 1996) and so influence development on multiple levels. The symptoms of PTSD are most usefully seen as the constricting result of chronic fear, and not as implying any kind of personal deficit. As the war literature tells us, heroes suffered from these symptoms as well as less valiant soldiers. Feminists also stress the role of environmental factors, such as blaming the victim and social isolation, that often exacerbate the negative effects of traumatic experience (Root, 1992). In general, these writers have a high regard for the healing power of connectedness with others and advocate a more balanced interpersonal, rather than almost exclusively intrapersonal, perspective on trauma, its aftermath, and treatment. Such a perspective fits well with the focus and theme of this book, which views individuals and their problems within the context of their most significant relationships.

Apart from the specific symptoms necessary for a formal diagnosis of PTSD, trauma can negatively impact every area of a person's life. When we listen to a story of trauma, we usually hear much more than the symptoms described in DSM-IV. We hear a story of problems in the following areas :

• *The regulation of emotion.* Survivors often vacillate between being carried away on the tide of compelling emotions or finding themselves numb and disconnected from any kind of feeling. The loss of ability to regulate anxiety and anger is perhaps the most significant general effect of traumatic experience (van der Kolk, 1996). So a policeman, recovering from an incident in which someone tried to stab him, "comes to" and finds himself shaking uncontrollably and hiding in his basement when his wife comes home early and slams the front door. A CSA survivor cannot control her rage with her young son. A client, talking about her mother leaving the room when her father began to hit her, becomes disoriented and "goes away" for a period of time, as she does when she becomes upset in interactions with her partner.

• *The survivor's relationship to his or her own body.* Survivors' pain often seems to be expressed by their bodies. As van der Kolk (1996) and other theorists note, "the body remembers." Somatization is part of the aftermath of trauma and may result in survivors feeling betrayed by their own bodies. Thus, a client describing her rape by her father to her spouse for the first time suddenly cannot move her legs; she is paralyzed. Sexual dysfunction and a general inability to take pleasure in their bodies is also common in trauma survivors.

• *The coping mechanisms* aimed at controlling the echoes of trauma become destructive in and of themselves. A client stops eating because this seems to dampen her anxiety and her rage. A client cuts her genitals and arms to end her periods of dissociation and numbness. A client attempts suicide to "get off the merry-go-round" of nightmares and feeling numb.

• Trauma impacts *the key cognitive schemas about the meaning of life* and hope for the future and so interferes with goal setting. Assumptions of justice and personal efficacy are shattered and lost.

• *Relationships with other people* are colored by mistrust and a sense of isolation and estrangement. Terry, a CSA survivor, told her husband in couple therapy, "You are a stranger; you live in a world without ghosts and demons. I am on another planet."

• *The survivor's sense of self* is often damaged and infused with shame and self-denigration. Survivors tend to blame and denigrate themselves for what has happened to them, and those closest to them often unwittingly magnify this response. A partner may, for example, minimize what has occurred to the survivor because he or she does not understand the nature of the trauma and may feel overwhelmed by the spouse's distress.

THE TRAUMA TRAP

How does a couple therapist who has been trained in systems theory and in general humanistic individual approaches to therapy, as many couple therapists have, make sense of trauma and its effects? Each of the preceding elements is problematic enough in itself. It is also helpful to think about how they link with and perpetuate each other. They become part of a process, an *absorbing inner state and a corresponding way of engaging with the world,* whereby, after a while, everything leads into a sense of darkness, helplessness, and hopelessness, and nothing leads out.

Survivors cannot count on being able to organize or regulate their own bodies or their emotional lives, and they cannot count on others. In fact, when our bodies and feelings are experienced as being out of our control, just being in touch with them seems dangerous. There is no touchstone, no firm ground where reality and the person's sense of self can be organized and integrated. After a while, helplessness and fear become self-perpetuating. A survivor once remarked, "I can't count on me. Panic can overwhelm me in a flash. And I am so watchful, so careful. Everything looks dangerous to me, even my spouse who loves me. At least, I know in my head he loves me, but . . . "

Another way to think about this phenomenon is that the effects of trauma reflect the essential nature of fear. Emotions are impulses to act, and fear is essentially a program for escape (Lang, 1979). When escape becomes impossible, however, fear itself can become aversive and debilitating and, ironically, renders coping ever more difficult. So Sarah, the victim of a past violent and abusive marriage, structures her life to deal with the terror that her violent partner aroused in her and her belief that he will one day come back and kill her. This terror lies in wait for her in dreams, in the shower where he used to attack, in any dark place. Thoughts of safety preoccupy her. She drives huge moving trucks so that no one can "see me, touch me, find me, or catch me." But still, when she sleeps, dreams of being pursued hijack her, as well as dreams of grief about all she lost in her abusive relationship. She is highly ambivalent about letting anyone close enough to hurt her and sets up constant tests for her present partner. She pushes him to get angry, and when he finally loses his temper, she declares him dangerous and untrustworthy. She has also reported that part of her believes what her abuser always told her, that she deserved his punishments, that she is flawed, weak, and shameful. There is only one organizing principle that Sarah can hold onto, and that is never to feel helpless and vulnerable again. The longer Sarah lives according to this principle, dealing with her fears by surrounding herself with steel, the more difficult it is for her to allow herself to be vulnerable and to face those fears. The more difficult it is, then, to let someone close enough to show her that not all men are like her abuser, that she is lovable and worthy of care, and even that she can allow herself to feel. Her tough, defensive stance limits the range of new experiences that might revise her view of the world, herself, and others.

The essential experience of trauma is one of helplessness and disorganization and constant attempts to ward off the memory of free fall. The struggle to fend off this sense of helplessness often becomes a victim's whole life. For example, a rape survivor's hypervigilance and mistrust of others leads her to isolate herself. In this isolation, images of the rape constantly arise and other people appear increasingly dangerous. The present is then framed and constructed in the image of the past.

Writers such as Shalev (1993) talk of trauma as a *trap*, in which one level of impairment prevents self-regulatory healing processes from occurring on other levels. Rather than thinking in terms of impairment, it seems that people create brilliant solutions or ways to defend themselves against the pain and chaos of trauma that allow them to survive the dragon's fire. Then they get stuck in trying to live encumbered by such defenses. The solutions become part of the problem and part of the toxicity of trauma. Bowlby (1973) explicitly related the dynamic concept of defense to the more systemic concept of organizing inner and outer realities into some kind of homeostasis. Such organization allows an individual to deal with one situation, but may then severely limit the options open to him or her in other situations. There are not many options when we face a dragon in the dark, and some of the options we choose make it difficult to then turn down other paths and find the light. The press of overwhelming emotions and images, for example, makes it hard for survivors to put words to their traumatic experiences and to structure them into sentences. It is easier to become numb or to split experiences into fragments. If a person cannot put words to an experience, however, it is hard to process and organize that experience. It is then even harder to tell it to another so that the other may understand and comfort. If a significant other cannot comfort, that person often becomes seen as the enemy. In the desperate darkness, if you are not with me, then you are against me.

RETRAUMATIZATION

It is also worth noting that victims of severe, intermittent trauma, especially in childhood, are likely to be retraumatized. One-half to one-third of women who experience sexual violence (rape or CSA) will be revictimized, and multiple victimizations lead to more severe stress responses (Folette, Polusny, Bechtle, & Naugle, 1996). Why does traumatization make people more vulnerable to retraumatization, and what does this tell us about the effects of trauma? This phenomenon is complex and can be seen from many angles. Let us address a few of them.

From a social learning perspective, victims have not learned how to protect themselves. They have learned that they are helpless and that passivity and numbing will at least ensure survival. As discussed earlier, survivors' methods of protecting themselves against past traumas, such as dissociating, often become problematic in and of themselves and make the survivors relatively defenseless in the face of new dangers. Survivors have often learned sexual behaviors that may have appeased perpetrators but now put these victims at risk. Handicapped by the effects of traumas already suffered, they may not be good at learning how to escape from new aversive situations (Chu, 1992).

From an attachment perspective, trauma victims may have no models of responsive, caring others and so may be unable to reach out and enlist support when they need it. Without the experience of secure attachment whereby a person feels valued and affirmed, it is difficult to develop positive self-esteem. It is then hard to fight against abuse if you feel that maybe you deserve it. It is even harder when you have little trust that others will support you in such a fight.

Trauma exacts a toll on the body. From a neurological point of view, there is evidence that traumatized women exhibit the neurological dysregulation characteristic of combat veterans (Stein, Yehuda, Koverola, & Hanna, 1997). Just one of the implications of this finding is that it is difficult for such individuals to use emotions as danger signals to prompt adaptive action. Chronic activation in brain systems seems to result in overreactions to nonemergencies and a freezing response in the face of real danger.

From the perspective of survivors, and sometimes their partners and communities, the road to retraumatization is often seen to lie in the deficits or even the masochism of the victim. It is important for therapists to have clear alternate models that do not result in blaming victims. In general, theoreticians with various perspectives seem to be espousing models similar to that described earlier, in which individuals narrow their lives to cope with terror and then become stuck and unable to adapt to new situations (Nichols, 1987). What is important for the couple therapist is that such conceptualizations promote respect for and the ability to connect with survivors and their secondarily traumatized partners. These conceptualizations are also more in tune with a systemic perspective and easily integrated with an interpersonal or relational approach than past models, which tended to be more intrapsychically oriented and pathologizing of survivors.

COPING WITH TRAUMA

What does it take to be able to fight the dragon well? There is no one who is immune to the fire of the dragon's breath. Writers such as Root (1992) remind us of the need to depathologize the effects of trauma, to recognize that all of us are vulnerable and that everyone has a breaking point. However, it is still worth considering: What gives us the best chance, not just at survival after trauma, but at being able to live a life out of the dragon's shadow?

All trauma theorists agree that first of all, a survivor needs a safe place to stand, a haven where this person feels protected from attack. Our health system offers safe, predictable environments, and medication can provide a rest from inner chaos. These supports can be invaluable. In the end, though, those who deal well with trauma are those who can turn to others for support. Therapists and members of survivors groups can offer that support, but it is important to remember that most often these people become, in a sense, stand-ins for attachment figures. The conclusion of numerous theorists and researchers over the years is that a secure attachment bond is the "primary defense against trauma induced psychopathology" (Finklehor & Browne, 1984). The best defense of all is to have a loved one stand beside you in the dark. Comfort and protection from those nearest to us is the path to resilience and healing that is wired in by evolution. This is the concept that is elaborated and illustrated in this book. However, it is important to consider the general factors that determine how any one of us will respond to traumatic events and what decides how resilient we will be.

Why do some trauma survivors suffer more debilitating effects than others? A review of the epidemiology of trauma suggests that on average about one-quarter of those exposed to trauma develop PTSD, although they may develop other problems or be given other diagnoses. There are some traumas so colossal in scope that most of those who are caught in them will continue to struggle with negative effects, often for the rest of their lives. But there are also individual differences in how people respond to trauma and how they deal with negative effects when they do arise.

The nature of the trauma obviously counts here. Norris (1992), in a study of 1,000 adults, found that 69% had experienced a traumatic stressor in their lives. The most common causes of PTSD in men seems to be combat or witnessing death or injury, whereas the most common cause of PTSD in women seems to be sexual assault. There is a consensus that trauma deliberately inflicted by one's fellow human beings has a more negative impact than natural disasters. Two decades after the war, 15% of combat troops in Vietnam were found to be suffering from PTSD and another 11% from partial PTSD (Kulka et al., 1990). Across studies, half or more of past political prisoners exhibited PTSD, and almost half of the women who experienced sexual assault were diagnosed with PTSD, although many of these women also improved over time. Substantial rates of PTSD have also been found among psychiatric patients and in accident victims such as burn patients. Furthermore, victims develop a range of disorders such as major depression and anxiety disorders, often together with partial symptoms of PTSD. In general, there is evidence that the importance of traumatic events as a cause of psychological symptoms has never been fully recognized (McFarlane & Girolamo, 1996; Read, 1997).

Victims of CSA particularly have been identified as being prone to DESNOS (disorders of extreme stress not otherwise specified) or complex PTSD (Zlotnick, et al., 1996). This categorization is intended to recognize the personality changes that occur as people, often traumatized at a young age by those they depend on, attempt to adapt to living with the aftereffects of such trauma. All trauma disrupts the victim's sense of self and how he or she makes sense of the world; however, this result is particularly likely when trauma is inflicted on young children by those they depend on most. These victims are more apt to have a range of dissociative symptoms and seem to be particularly likely to be self-denigrating and to inflict harm on themselves. It is probably more adaptive, at least in the short run, to believe that you are to blame and deserve cruel treatment, than that you are helpless and dependent on people who wish you harm. Such survivors are also likely to display anger and hostility to others and to be labeled with borderline personality disorders. They are also prone to substance abuse in an attempt to regulate their distress.

Apart from the nature of the trauma, the characteristics of the survivor and the nature of the recovery environment play a part in determining who will suffer long-term effects. In terms of the characteristics of survivors, a key factor seems to be the meaning people give to their traumatic experiences. Trauma seems to be particularly pernicious when such an experience defines the survivor's sense of self and leads to a sense of personal unworthiness. Stigma and self-blame have been found to mediate adult adjustment in child abuse survivors (Coffey, Leitenberg, Henning, & Turner, 1996). Another factor is the victim's sense of efficacy or belief in the ability to control what happens to him or her. Studies of inescapable shock in animals found that those who had previously experienced being able to escape, thus exerting some control over their environment, were more resilient to future shocks. An internal locus of control that promotes active coping in the face of danger and a sense of optimism seems to create resilience in those who are sexually abused as children. Some victims can then create a framework for themselves in which they can maintain a sense of control over their future (Himelein & McElrath, 1996). Resilient victims also tend not to blame themselves for the abuse (Valentine & Feinauer, 1993). Perhaps such victims had the experience of a secure attachment figure that validated their experience and helped them maintain their self-esteem. The capacity to preserve a social connection to others also seems to protect people from trauma. Those who are able to disclose the trauma, and so process it and elicit the support of others in finding meaning in their ordeal, do better as well.

HEALING FROM TRAUMA

The trauma literature appears to be clear and unanimous concerning the nature of the recovery environment that promotes healing from traumatic experience. The functioning of burn patients was predicted best by the amount of social support they received, not the extent of their injuries or facial disfigurement (Perry, Difade, Musngi, Frances, & Jacobsberg, 1992). The literature on the positive difference social support makes to those who have experienced traumatic stress is vast. Recently, however, it has become clear that to be resilient in the face of trauma, people need not just friends and a sense of community, but close attachment bonds. The quality of such bonds is clearly linked with the ability to regulate emotions and develop an integrated concept of self, both of which have been associated with resilience in later life (Mikulincer, 1995; Sroufe, 1996). Those of us who have known at least one secure attachment as children seem to have more resources to fight the dragon should he come for us. Those who have a secure sense of attachment as adults are not only more resilient (Mikulincer, Florian, & Weller, 1993), but have a safe haven that promotes healing if trauma does occur.

On the other hand, a lack of secure attachment makes us more vulnerable to traumatic stress. For children who are severely abused and who develop what is termed disorganized or fearful-avoidant attachment patterns, characterized by approach–avoidance contact with attachment figures, both inner and outer worlds are characterized by chaos. They are unable to create a safe, stable place to stand. So when another dragon appears, they are more vulnerable and less able to fight effectively. Such children also, by necessity, develop ways of coping that may perpetuate the effects of the original abuse and make them more vulnerable. The experience of childhood abuse is closely linked to the initiation of self-destructive behavior, but the lack of secure attachments seems to maintain such behavior (van der Kolk, 1996).

A GENERAL PERSPECTIVE ON TRAUMA

There are many approaches to understanding trauma. The main focus in this book is on using an interpersonally oriented intervention, couple therapy, to help survivors. It seems natural, then, that we look at trauma with a more interpersonal focus. The symptoms of PTSD in DSM-

IV focus on intrapsychic rather than interpersonal phenomena. To extend this viewpoint, it seems useful to consider the general theoretical frameworks that support a more interpersonal view of trauma and its effects:

- Social constructionist perspectives are now emphasizing the impact of the social environment on how we construe reality. The meaning we give to events is partly determined by social context. Most rapes are unreported because to be raped is still to be shamed, and to accuse one's attacker is most often to be retraumatized in a court of law. To come home from World War II and be recognized as a savior was a different experience from that most Canadian Vietnam veterans had when they came home to Canada and felt compelled to keep their participation in the war a secret.

- New feminist approaches to psychology, such as that of the Stone Center theorists (Jordan et al., 1991), emphasize that identity formation and maintenance involve relational events that take place between people rather than inside the head.

- Attachment theory is increasingly being used to understand how intrapsychic issues such as affect regulation and information processing are formed and maintained by social relationships, particularly with those we depend on. Personality, as construed by Sullivan (1953) many years ago and by modern attachment theorists such as Sroufe (1996), *is* the way we habitually engage other people.

All of these perspectives can be viewed as consonant with the systems perspective (von Bertalanffy, 1956; Erdman & Caffrey, in press) that the family therapy field has bequeathed to couple therapists. This perspective promotes a focus on the present and on the process of interaction between intimates. It does not preclude a focus on how individuals actively construct their inner emotional worlds (Johnson, 1998). In fact, it is in the bridging of self and system, the within and between, that couple interventions for survivors can have the most impact. When working with traumatized couples and with individual trauma survivors, I assume that key interactions with others create emotional states and ways of construing reality and that these states and construals, in turn, structure key interactions. My colleagues and I are focused on discovering how key interactions call up and maintain traumatic inner realities. We are also seeking to determine how these realities structure and maintain particular kinds of engagement with others in a reciprocal cycle. Most of the traumas our clients bring to therapy are what Herman (1992) calls "violations of human connection," and in these in particular, engagement with others is the dragon's cave. Dealing with key issues, such as how ways of regulating affect and defining the self can prevent healing and perpetuate the effects of trauma, always involves working with survivors' relationships.

THE TREATMENT OF TRAUMA

The couple therapist who works with traumatized couples needs a general knowledge of trauma interventions, most of which have been elaborated within the framework of individual therapy. In many traumatized couples who seek a couple therapist, the survivor is already engaged in some form of individual therapy or group treatment. The couple therapist must be aware of the total treatment plan and where the survivor stands in relation to his or her trauma, so as to integrate couple interventions with other therapies. Occasionally, a couple will seek a couple therapist first, or as part of the treatment for associated problems such as depression, and the survivor's trauma to this point will have been untouched or even unrecognized. The couple therapist may then provide the first orientation to coping with trauma for the survivor. Couple therapists also have to deal actively with trauma symptoms, such as the shame that promotes interpersonal withdrawal, just as the individual therapist does, albeit in a different modality. Even if clients have individual therapists, occasionally a couple therapist may also conduct some individual sessions to focus on a specific aspect of the traumatic experience that seems to be blocking progress in the couple sessions. Often, however, survivors request couple therapy when intrusive symptoms have begun to abate and emotional detachment or estrangement from others becomes the most pertinent problem. Even then, when a survivor begins to risk emotional engagement with a spouse, intrusive symptoms may temporarily recur. For all of these reasons, a couple therapist who deals with trauma needs to know about general interventions for the aftereffects of trauma and how to deal with PTSD symptoms when they arise. It is safe to assume that the vast majority of survivors will need some form of individual therapy *and* that, in all likelihood, they will also need couple therapy, group therapy, or both. Different modalities may inform and potentiate each other. They may deal with different aspects of survivors' problems. They may also deal with core issues, such as negative definitions of self, in different contexts, where new routes to change become accessible.

INDIVIDUAL THERAPY FOR TRAUMA

For the reasons discussed previously, we now briefly consider the role of individual therapy in treatment of trauma survivors. Cognitive-behavioral, psychodynamic, and humanistic experiential models have all been applied to trauma survivors, and they have also been applied in group formats. Cognitive-behavioral approaches, particularly prolonged *in vivo* and imaginal exposure to reduce fear and anxiety, have been found to be effective in reducing specific symptoms of PTSD, particularly for traumas such as rape (Foa & Rothbaum, 1998). Experiential interventions (Paivio & Nieuwenhuis, 2001) and more dynamic therapies (Brom & Kleber, 1989; Gersons & Carlier, 1994) have also been found to reduce anxiety and improve functioning. However, most individual therapists seem to use an eclectic assortment of interventions (Blake, 1993), perhaps because clients most often do not come to therapy simply to reduce specific symptoms. They come to take their lives back from trauma and address more general issues such as depression, somatization, and the inability to trust others. Specific intrusive and hyperarousal symptoms generally seem to improve after techniques such as flooding or imaginal exposure, but constrictive symptoms such as numbing and social withdrawal do not necessarily improve and seem to be harder to modify. Specific techniques generally seem to work best for clients dealing with single traumatic events rather than repeated abuse. For treatment of survivors of childhood sexual abuse, who are more likely to have complex PTSD, several general treatment models have been proposed (Courtois, 1988; McCann & Pearlman, 1990). However, only two clinical trials of specific interventions have been conducted with these clients, in spite of the voluminous literature on treating individual survivors that has emerged over the last few years. These trials were conducted by Alexander and her colleagues (Alexander, Neimeyer, Follette, Moore, & Harter, 1989) and Paivio and Nieuwenhuis (2001). There seems to be a consensus, across all models of therapy, that the presence of PTSD reflects primarily an impairment in the emotional processing of the traumatic experience (Foa & Rothbaum, 1998; van der Kolk, McFarlane, & Weisaeth, 1996).

Two basic goals of trauma treatment are identified repeatedly by clinicians ascribing to all models of individual therapy. The first is affect regulation, specifically, the taming of fear and anger. The second is the creation of new meanings that allow the traumatic experience to be integrated into a positive and empowered sense of self. It is interesting, however, that even if the goals of therapy are framed in intrapsychic terms, clinicians generally agree that the "success of treatment depends on the patient's ability to tolerate intimacy, in other words, the patient's ability to trust another person with his or her helplessness and pain" (Turner, McFarlane, & van der Kolk, 1996). *Success in helping the survivor recast his or her intrapsychic world depends on the creation of new interpersonal connections.* This is necessary for the process of intrapsychic change and is also, although often left in the background, a major goal of therapy.

One of the strengths of the couple therapy modality is that, in such therapy sessions, survivors make new interpersonal connections not only with a therapist but in their ongoing intimate relationships. Herman (1992) stresses that both individual therapy, to desensitize traumatic memory, and group therapy, to create reconnection with others, are probably necessary for full recovery. This book stresses couple therapy, rather than group therapy, as the main arena for reconnection. Herman notes that in many studies of stress and captivity in war, such as in concentration camps, the pair rather than the individual proved to be the basic unit of survival. Such a bond thus seems to be a more potent natural healing context than a treatment group. Thus, therapeutic groups and individual interventions may have a limited impact on recovery if pair bond dynamics are not also actively addressed. As Bateson pointed out (1972), "When you separate mind from the structure in which it is immanent—such as human relationships . . . you embark . . . on fundamental error" (p. 493). Consider a study of how people coped with the death of a child. Typically, women became depressed and men withdrew into tasks. These men perhaps did not know how to respond to their wives' grief and feared losing control. The women then suffered a double loss. Yet if the husband stayed engaged and the couple faced their grief together, the relationship improved and grief was dealt with constructively (Videka-Sherman, 1982; Videka-Sherman & Lieberman, 1985).

RECOVERY FROM TRAUMA

What constitutes recovery from trauma? It is surely more than the abatement of particular symptoms. It is also more specific than a kind of global mental health that we all aspire to but may never reach. Harvey (1996) suggests an interpersonal ecological model that views health in terms of the fit between an individual and his or her context. At best, this fit reduces isolation, fosters social competence, and supports connection with others and positive coping. She suggests that recovery involves the following:

1. Authority over the remembering process and the creation of a meaningful life story in which traumatic memories have a context, rather than simply being encoded as vivid sensations and memories.
2. The integration of memory and affect. Emotion without memory is disorienting, terrifying, or both, and memory without affect, as Breuer and Freud (1955) noted, produces no result because there is no closure.
3. Affect tolerance. The individual is no longer subject to overwhelming arousal, undue alarm, defensive numbing, and dangerous impulses.
4. Symptom mastery and healthy coping.
5. Self-esteem and self-cohesion. Shame and self-blame are relinquished.
6. The creation of new meaning, which is assigned to and transforms the trauma.
7. The creation of safe attachment and the ability to trust others.

In the journey toward recovery in individual treatment, most clinicians identify stages similar to the three stages described by McCann and Pearlman (1990): stabilization, working through the trauma and building self and relational capacities, and consolidation and integration. These stages are discussed in some detail in the following sections. Chapter 5 presents a couple therapy model including these stages.

STAGE 1. STABILIZATION

Fear must be held in check so that a survivor can catch his or her breath, look around, and begin to give words to the "speechless terror" that is often expressed only in somatic symptoms. In fight or flight situations immediate survival is the issue, not new learning and the piecing together of alternative responses. Unfortunately, survivors may constantly be lapsing into fight, flight, or freeze states because almost anything turns on their inner alarms. The first task recognized by all trauma therapists is to create a safe place where the dragon is held at bay and the survivor is not always on the verge of being overwhelmed. Because survivors experience not just the outer, but also their inner, world as a danger zone, they first need a safe haven to even begin focusing on their inner world as it unfolds in the present moment. The creation of a trusting alliance with the therapist, a factor found to be consistently associated with successful outcome in psychotherapy, is crucial in working with trauma survivors.

Other elements that most therapists include at this stage of therapy, which should also be addressed in couple therapy, for the benefit of the partner as well as the survivor, are the following:

- education about trauma symptoms
- naming problematic affective states and the action tendencies they evoke
- outlining positive ways to begin to regulate these emotions and any associated somatic responses
- naming and reducing any negative methods of affect regulation, such as social withdrawal or substance abuse, that the survivor habitually uses

STAGE 2. RESTRUCTURING BONDS: THE BUILDING OF SELF AND RELATIONAL CAPACITIES

The elements included here may be dealt with in different ways by therapists using different models of intervention and across different modalities, such as individual and couple therapies. These elements are:

- Owning and integrating memories and forming them into a coherent narrative. When the survivor can gather fragmented images, body sensations, and thoughts, put them together in a context, and create a story of helplessness survived, this evokes a sense of mastery. The survivor becomes the author of his or her story rather than the puppet of traumatic events. This objective may be achieved with the use of many different techniques, such as cognitive therapy, desensitization, or supportive psychotherapy, all of which seem to be somewhat effective (Resnick, Jordan, Girelli, Hunter, & Marhoerer-Dvorak, 1988). The central point is that the client confronts the trauma, but this time experiences some control and mastery rather than overwhelming helplessness.
- Owning and tolerating the powerful emotional responses, such

as fear and rage, that accompany trauma cues and images, so that emotions can be regulated and linked to specific meaning schemes.

- Making explicit and dealing with the implications of the trauma story for the survivor's sense of self. For example, the therapist helps the survivor verbalize and confront shame and self-hate and so reformulate the meaning of trauma experiences as they relate to his or her identity.

- Dealing with the grief and loss that arise as the survivor is able to piece together and make explicit the story of the trauma and the price of survival.

- Determining the nature of the survivor's relationships with others and supporting attempts to make new kinds of interpersonal connections. As van der Kolk (1996) states, "Treatment cannot address past trauma unless its echoes and replays in current relationships are also vigorously addressed." In individual therapy these echoes are presumably addressed through examining the client's interactions with the therapist and through discussing the client's relationships outside therapy. Positive relationships not only foster engagement in the other tasks included in this list, but provide an antidote to traumatic experience and restore hope that life can be worth living.

STAGE 3. CONSOLIDATION AND INTEGRATION

In all therapies, there is a stage concerned with consolidating the gains made in treatment and supporting the survivor to begin a new way of life in which the trauma experience becomes background rather than the client's dominant life theme. In successful therapy, survivors now have new ways to tame and manage emotional states, more positive views of the self and others, and frames for the trauma that allow for hope and efficacy in their lives. The techniques involved in individual therapy for survivors are numerous—flooding, rapid eye movement desensitization, insight, and cognitive restructuring, among others. They all require a secure relationship with the therapist, which may, in itself, be difficult to achieve. There is evidence that some techniques have greater impact on particular problems. For example, more dynamic expressive therapies may affect avoidance symptoms more effectively than desensitization techniques that primarily target anxiety (Brom & Kleber, 1989).

The approach to individual treatment that best fits with the main model of couple therapy described in this book is experiential therapy. This approach focuses on the processing of affect (Greenberg et al., 1993) and its integration into new meaning schemes and narratives. Experiental therapy has recently been formulated into a clear set of techniques and short-term change processes (Paivio & Nieuwenhuis, 2001; Paivio & Shimp, 1998). The main theoretical orientation toward close relationships used in this book, attachment theory, is now also being used by a number of individual therapists as a framework to direct interventions in complex stress disorders that arise from incest experiences (Alexander & Andersen, 1994).

Any therapy that attempts to help trauma survivors make significant changes in their lives must address many problems. For the vast majority of clients, such treatment involves much more than the desensitization of traumatic memories in individual therapy. Van der Kolk (1996) notes that, for survivors, recovery is essentially an *interpersonal* process that changes survivors' relationships with others: "Effective psychotherapy needs to address specifically how the trauma has affected people's sense of self-efficacy, their capacity for trust and intimacy, their ability to negotiate their personal needs, and their ability to feel empathy for other people. . . . This is often best accomplished in a group therapy setting" (p. 432). This description of the process of therapy fits with my colleagues' and my own clinical experience. However, support by people outside therapy groups has been found to be more closely related to symptom relief than support offered by group members (Coble, Gantt, & Mallinckrodt, 1996). Moreover, a recent study of group therapy for CSA survivors found that group therapy seemed to have an impact on some intrapsychic problems, but no effect on the interpersonal problems in the clients' lives outside the group (Saxe & Johnson, 1999). The rest of this book is dedicated to the idea that for many adult survivors of trauma, the essential elements in the process of change, as outlined earlier, are best addressed in their natural context. This context is the emotional connection and attachment of the pair bond, and the treatment modality that addresses that bond most directly, couple therapy.

Chapter 3

Attachment and Trauma

Emotional attachment is probably the primary
protection against feelings of helplessness and
meaninglessness.
—MCFARLANE and VAN DER KOLK (1996, p. 24)

A sense of felt security with a loved one increases a person's ability to tolerate and cope with traumatic experience. The attachment system is evolution's way of maximizing survival in a dangerous world, a world in which a person cannot survive alone. Secure attachment, as formulated by John Bowlby (1969), provides a *safe haven* and a *secure base* from which to explore and learn about the world. Secure attachment creates resilience in the face of terror and helplessness and a natural arena for healing. Isolation and a lack of secure attachment, on the other hand, add to our vulnerability, exacerbate traumatic events, and are actually wounding in themselves. It is also hard to develop an integrated, confident sense of self without secure connections to significant others. As Merleau Ponty states, "I borrow myself from others: man is a mirror for man."

Attachment theory is a systemic theory that looks at people in the context of their habitual interactions with those who are most important to them (Johnson & Best, in press). Both attachment theory, which offers the couple and family therapist a theory of intimate relationships, and the recent trauma literature encourage clinicians to look at people in context. Both take us away from personal deficit models. Attachment theory encourages us to look at how habitual ways of engaging others structure our inner world. The trauma literature focuses on how our ways of coping with difficult events also structure our world and how we engage with others. John Bowlby was arguably the first family therapist. In 1949 he published a paper describing how he interviewed parents about their childhood experiences, in the presence of their troubled children, to achieve clinical change. He was trained as a psychoanalyst, but he believed in the power of the environment and shared ideas with Bertalanffy, the father of systems theory, and primate researchers like Harry Harlow and Robert Hinde. Bowlby insisted on looking at what occurs within *and* between people and at how each person affects the other. He believed that mental health professionals neglected the role of real environmental trauma in the genesis of emotional and mental health problems. He also believed that the effects of such trauma were then perpetuated by the need for inner defenses, such as the suppression of negative affect, if no outer supports were available. Bowlby offers the trauma therapist and the couple therapist an interpersonal theory that addresses and integrates how individuals construct and maintain a sense of self and relatedness to others and how they deal with danger and stress.

Isolation and a lack of secure connection to others undermine a person's ability to deal with traumatic experience. Conversely, secure emotional connections with significant others offer a powerful antidote to traumatic experience (Johnson, in press). How does safe attachment to another provide an antidote to the ravages of trauma? Consider how the effects of trauma and the effects of safe attachment, as defined by Bowlby and other recent attachment theorists (Bowlby, 1969, 1973, 1980, 1988; Cassidy & Shaver, 1999) mesh and contrast. The following table contrasts the effects of trauma with the protective effects of a secure connectedness with attachment figures.

Traumatic experience	Secure attachment
Floods us with physical fear/helplessness.	Soothes and comforts.
Colors the world as dangerous/ unpredictable.	Offers a safe haven.
Creates overwhelming emotional chaos.	Promotes affect regulation/integration.
Threatens a cohesive sense of self.	Promotes personality integration.
Assaults self-efficacy and a sense of control.	Promotes confidence/trust in self and others.
Scrambles the ability to engage fully in the present, and so to adapt to new situations.	Promotes openness to experience, risk taking, and new learning.

The contrasts presented here appear to hold whether we are talking about the trauma of physical separation, alienation and grief in disrupted attachments (attachment injuries; see Chapter 10), single traumas such as accidents and rape, the traumas of war, or traumas such as childhood sexual abuse. Civilians who experience secure attachments are more resilient in situations of war, such as missile attacks (Mikulincer et al., 1993). A significant proportion of clients identified as having borderline personality disorders, most of whom are survivors of childhood sexual abuse (CSA), improve substantially in later life if they find a positive attachment relationship with an understanding other (Stone, 1990).

Whereas secure attachment protects us, insecure attachment, unfortunately, often intensifies and perpetuates the effects of traumatic experience. If trauma is actually inflicted by such attachment figures, this tends not only to intensify the negative effects, but also to contaminate future connections with other attachment figures and interfere with the natural processes of growth and healing.

INTRODUCTION TO ATTACHMENT THEORY

The 10 central tenets of attachment theory are as follows:

1. *Attachment is an innate motivating force.* Seeking and maintaining contact with significant others is an innate, primary motivating principle in human beings across the life span. Dependency, which has been pathologized in our culture (Bowlby, 1988), is an innate part of being human rather than a childhood trait that we outgrow.

2. *Secure dependence complements autonomy.* According to attachment theory, there is no such thing as complete independence from others or overdependence (Bretherton & Munholland, 1999). There is only effective or ineffective dependence. Secure dependence fosters autonomy and self-confidence. Secure dependence and autonomy are two sides of the same coin, rather than dichotomies. The more securely connected we are, the more separate and different we can be.

3. *Attachment offers a safe haven.* Such contact is an innate survival mechanism. The presence of an attachment figure, which usually means parents, children, spouses, and lovers, provides comfort and security, and the perceived inaccessibility of such a figure creates distress. Positive attachments create *a safe haven* that offers a buffer against the

effects of stress and uncertainty and an optimal context for the continuing development of the personality.

4. *Attachment offers a secure base.* Secure attachment also provides a *secure base* from which individuals can explore their universe and most adaptively respond to their environment. The presence of such a base encourages exploration and a cognitive openness to new information. It promotes the confidence necessary to risk, learn, and continually update models of self and the world.

5. *Accessibility and responsiveness build bonds.* The building blocks of secure bonds are emotional accessibility and responsiveness. It is emotional engagement that is crucial. In attachment terms, any response (even anger) is better than none. If there is no engagement, no emotional responsiveness, the message from the attachment figure is "Your signals do not matter, and there is no connection between us."

6. *Fear and uncertainty activate attachment needs.* When an individual is threatened—by traumatic events, the negative aspects of everyday life such as illness, or an assault on the security of the attachment bond itself—emotions arise, attachment needs for comfort and connection become particularly salient and compelling, and attachment behaviors, such as proximity seeking, are activated. Proximity to a loved one is an inbuilt emotion-regulation device.

7. *The process of separation distress is predictable.* If attachment behaviors fail to evoke comforting contact and responsiveness from an attachment figure, a prototypical process of angry protest, clinging, depression, and despair occurs, culminating eventually in detachment. Depression is a natural response to loss of connection. Bowlby (1973) distinguished between the anger of hope and the anger of despair, which becomes desperate and coercive.

8. *A finite number of insecure forms of engagement can be identified.* The number of ways human beings have to deal with the unresponsiveness of attachment figures is limited. There are only so many ways of coping with a negative answer to the question, "Can I depend on you when I need you?" Attachment responses to such answers seem to be organized along two dimensions, anxiety and avoidance (Fraley & Waller, 1998). When the connection with an irreplaceable other is threatened but not yet severed, the attachment system may go into overdrive. Attachment behaviors become heightened and intense as anxious clinging, pursuit, and even aggressive attempts to obtain a response from the loved one escalate. The second strategy for dealing with the lack of safe emotional engagement, especially when hope for respon-

siveness has been lost, is to suppress attachment needs, focus on tasks, and limit or avoid distressing emotional engagement with the attachment figure. These two strategies, anxious clinging and detached avoidance, can develop into habitual styles of engagement with intimate others. These strategies were first identified in experimental separations and reunions of mothers and infants (Ainsworth, Blehar, Waters, & Wall, 1978). Some infants were able to modulate their distress on separation, to make reassuring contact with the mother when she returned, and then, confident of her responsiveness if she was needed, to return to exploration and play. These infants were viewed as securely attached. Others became extremely distressed on separation and clung to or expressed anger to the mother on reunion. They were difficult to soothe and were viewed as anxiously attached. Another group showed signs of physiological distress but exhibited little emotion at separation or reunion. They focused on tasks and activities and were seen as avoidantly attached. These styles are "self-maintaining patterns of social interaction and emotion regulation strategies" (Shaver & Clarke, 1994, p. 119). They echo the general display modes for emotion that Ekman and Friesen (1975) identify: exaggerating, substituting one feeling for another, as when we focus on anger rather than fear, and minimizing. Although these habitual forms of engagement can be modified by new relationships, they can also mold current relationships and so become self-perpetuating. They involve specific behavioral responses to regulate emotions and protect the self from rejection and abandonment, and cognitive schemas or working models of the self and the other. In the attachment literature the term *styles*, which implies individual characteristics, is often used interchangeably with the term *strategies*, which implies behavior that is more context-specific. The term *forms of engagement*, coined by Sroufe (1996), can be used to further stress the interpersonal nature of this concept.

9. *Attachment involves working models of the self and the other.* As stated earlier, attachment strategies reflect ways of processing and dealing with emotion. Some spouses catastrophize and complain when they feel rejected; some become silent for days. Bowlby (1969) outlined the cognitive content of the representations of the self and the other that are inherent in these responses. Secure attachment is characterized by a working model of a self that is worthy of love and care and is confident and competent. And, indeed, research has found secure attachment to be associated with self-efficacy (Mikulincer, 1995). Securely attached people, who believe others will be responsive when needed, tend to

have working models of others as dependable and worthy of trust. These models of the self and the other, distilled from a thousand interactions, then became expectations and biases that are carried forward into new relationships. They are not simple cognitive schemas. They involve goals, beliefs, and strategies, and they are heavily infused with emotion. *Working models are formed, elaborated, maintained, and, most important for the couple therapist, changed through emotional communication.*

10. *Isolation and loss are inherently traumatizing.* Perhaps most significant for the couple therapist is that attachment theory is a theory of trauma. Bowlby began his career as a health professional by studying maternal deprivation and separation and its effects on children. Attachment theory describes and explains the trauma of deprivation, loss, rejection, and abandonment by those we need most and its enormous effect on us. Bowlby (1973) viewed these traumatic stressors, and the isolation that ensued, as having tremendous impact on personality formation and a person's ability to deal with other stresses in life. He believed that when someone is confident that a loved one will be there when needed, "a person will be much less prone to either intense or chronic fear than will an individual who has no such confidence" (p. 406). The couple therapist knows about the stress of deprivation and separation well. It is an essential part of the ongoing drama of "ordinary" marital distress. Clients often speak of such distress in terms of trauma, that is, in life and death terms (Johnson, 1997), and it is clearly related to symptoms such as depression and hypervigilance. In complex PTSD, we see that survivors cannot use current relationships to regulate fears and help them heal their wounds because specific, past violations of human connection often contaminate their current relationships. For the victim of childhood sexual abuse, the antidote of safe attachment is most often out of reach and the effects of trauma are then maintained or continually amplified.

Patterned responses, whether they are called attachment strategies, attachment styles, or simply habitual forms of engagement, are identified in the attachment literature. Habitual strategies for engaging with others and construing attachment situations affect the way people deal with traumatic experiences. These strategies or styles may best be thought of as ongoing constructions. Such constructions may be more or less rigidly structured and more or less open to revision. They involve ways of dealing with emotions, working models of the self and the other that bias perception and color meaning, and predispositions to particular behavioral responses in interactions. They are perhaps like individual scripts for a play; however, there is always another actor in this play, the attachment figure. This actor's responses and scripts also influence the form the play will take and how the individual structures particular scenes. Working models can and do change in new relationships (Davila, Karney, & Bradbury, 1999). In fact, to be optimally useful, they must be constantly revised and kept up to date.

As a couple therapist, I tend to think of working models as continually being formed and reformed in present interactions, with past scripts as background reference points. *The reason working models and the associated engagement strategies remain stable, when they do, is that they are actively constructed, enacted, and confirmed in present relationships.* Some other theorists tend to focus more on the predictive power of the past and how past childhood attachment models determine present relationships. However, all agree that these strategies play a part in organizing present interactions, which can, in turn, mitigate or intensify, confirm or revise a person's habitual strategy. Thus, a trauma survivor can, as a result of past experience, find it difficult to reach for a partner's help when a flashback occurs. The survivor then faces the dragon alone and again confirms that others are untrustworthy. When that person does manage to evoke the partner's caring at such times, however, new ways of engaging in such relationships and conceptualizing the self and others open up to the survivor. In change events in couple therapy (Johnson, 1996, 1999) the therapist can see the new ways of dealing with emotions and attachment needs and the new ways of perceiving the self and the other that follow from new steps in the attachment dance.

Insecure styles or strategies are not pathological; they are all adaptive at times. In certain situations, numbing ourselves and minimizing our attachment needs will maximize the responsiveness of a volatile and abusive attachment figure and protect us from the pain of frequent rejection. Such styles are best thought of as adaptive secondary strategies for maintaining the proximity of less-than-responsive caregivers. They become risk factors, however, when they become rigid and closed and pull strongly for particular confirming responses from a partner. In such cases, when a partner responds in a way that disconfirms a person's biases, these responses may not be recognized or trusted. So when Emma, an anxiously attached wife attempts to coerce her partner into increased responsiveness, but does not trust his response and so discounts it when he gives it, she alienates him further. Certain styles can block new learning and so become self-fulfilling prophecies. Trauma survivors may need very little confirmation in present interactions with partners to evoke negative attachment models from the past. Yet attachment strategies seem to change when people have compelling emotional experiences of comfort and connection that disconfirm past fears and biases and allow working models to be expanded and elaborated (Collins & Read, 1994).

These strategies seem to predict key relationship behaviors, such as responses to conflict and responses to seeking and giving support. Those with secure styles are generally happier and more able to reach out for and provide support (Simpson, 1990; Simpson, Rholes, & Nelligan, 1992; Simpson, Rholes, & Phillips, 1996). They have closer and more trusting relationships, can better acknowledge and communicate their needs, and are less likely to be verbally aggressive or withdraw during problem solving (Senchak & Leonard, 1992). Avoidant partners' relationships tend to be distant and untrusting. They withdraw particularly when they or their partners are vulnerable, and avoid depending on others. Anxious partners' relationships are often full of hypervigilance, jealousy, and worry about abandonment. Partnerships in which both partners are avoidant or anxious are rare, presumably because they are difficult to sustain. Clinicians have noted that in the office of the couple therapist, anxious-avoidant couplings seem commonplace. Research suggests that partnerships including at least one secure partner are more harmonious and have fewer conflictual interactions (Cohn, Silver, Cowan, Cowan, & Pearson, 1992).

ATTACHMENT THEORY AND THE QUALITY OF ADULT LOVE RELATIONSHIPS

Attachment theory is a "theory of love and its central place in human life" (Karen, 1998, p. 3). This theory provides a map to adult love relationships and how they become distressed. It also helps us understand how positive, close connections allow us to cope with dragons and dark places, so it is particularly relevant to truamatized couples. However, it took nearly two decades since Bowlby published Volume 1 of his attachment trilogy (1969) for his theory to be applied to adult love relationships by social psychologists (e.g., Hazan & Shaver, 1987) and clinical psychologists (e.g., Johnson, 1986). Couple therapy, in general, has long been in need of a theory of love. Any clinical intervention requires a map delineating what constitutes happiness and distress and the various routes people take to get to these destinations. Without such a theory, how do we know which changes will really make a difference? Individual therapists need a model of individual personality and growth, and couple therapists need a model of close relationships. Fortunately, there is now a large and growing body of literature addressing adult love from an attachment perspective (Bartholomew & Perlman, 1994; Cassidy & Shaver, 1999; Shaver & Hazan, 1993; Sperling & Berman, 1994).

Attachment theorists have divided adult bonds into three elements: attachment, caring, and sexuality (Hazan & Shaver, 1994). They have surmised that it takes about 2 years, on average, for a romantic affiliation to become a full attachment bond. Some have suggested that, in fact, caring and sexuality are properly seen as part of attachment and that attachment integrates these other elements. Sexuality in particular is a route to pair bonding. It seems that we are truly bonded only with those we touch.

As we go into the new millenium, attachment theory offers couple therapists not only a well-researched theory of adult love relationships, but one that dovetails with the recent research on the nature of marital distress by John Gottman and his colleagues (Gottman, 1994; Gottman, Coan, Carrere, & Swanson, 1998; Pasch & Bradbury, 1998). These authors stress the crucial importance of emotional engagement and comforting, soothing interactions in relationship definition. More is also being written about the impact of positive emotional bonds on mental and physical health, which relates to this attachment perspective. Close bonds are physiological regulators. Contact with those we love and depend on "tranquillizes the nervous system" (Schore, 1994). Moreover, an empirically validated treatment approach to couple therapy has evolved, using an attachment orientation (Johnson, Hunsley, Greenberg, & Schindler, 1999). This is emotionally focused couple therapy (EFT), which Les Greenberg and I developed in the early 1980s (Johnson, 1996). How this approach is adapted to partners with different attachment styles is explored elsewhere (Johnson & Whiffen, 1999).

It is perhaps important to note briefly some of the key criticisms of attachment theory that are relevant for the couple therapist. No theory is perfect or able to completely encompass the breadth and complexity of life. One criticism of attachment theory is that it does not take sufficient account of cultural differences. Although there are profound similarities in how the majority of families and couples create bonds (van IJzendoorn & Sagi, 1999), there are also differences in values and in how attachment needs are expressed (Rothbaum, Weisz, Pott, Miyake, & Morelli, 2000). Consider, for example, a certain couple from India. The husband suffered from PTSD after imprisonment and torture and was torn about whom he should turn to for comfort: his wife, whom he was still getting to know after an arranged marriage, or his mother, who made him the center of her life. Some cultures may also foster physical touch and holding for comfort more than others. In clinical practice, no theory can substitute for an active exploration of and respect for the meaning system of particular clients. The classification of forms of engagement or styles in attachment theory, although offering the therapist and clients a useful template, are still approximations and abstractions. They "miss much of the poetry and texture" of individual lives (Karen, 1998, p. 439) and of individual stances in specific relationships. Thus it is more appropriate for the therapist to use the theory as a template rather than a formula. The therapist must also tune in to the uniqueness of each couple's relationship and each partner's way of constructing his or her experience of connection with loved ones.

There are other elements in relationships besides attachment, and although Bowlby asserted that he could not be faulted for being unable to study everything (Karen, 1998), there are some who question whether he pays enough attention to power dynamics and gender in relationships. For example, it has been observed that fewer men than women with PTSD come for couple therapy. Is this because women are socialized to be caregivers, more tolerant of problem behaviors, and more used to providing a safe haven in which such male survivors can heal? Attachment theory does, however, posit basic needs for accessibility and responsiveness in both men and women. The descriptions of the kinds of relationships promoted by gender-sensitive therapy (Haddock, Schindler Zimmerman, & MacPhee, 2000), which are characterized by mutuality, reciprocity, and interdependency, sound remarkably similar to secure bonds as described by attachment theorists.

Finally, the descriptions of interventions in Bowlby's work seem to focus greatly on the formation of individual insight. Thus, the extension of this theory into the realm of clinical intervention is still developing. Certainly, this theory can tell the couple therapist what to attend to, what goals to pursue, and how to understand certain key behaviors, but Bowlby's original formulations of attachment theory cannot tell the therapist exactly how best to shift a couple toward, for example, increased accessibility. Let us now return to the main focus of this book, attachment responses and healing from trauma.

ATTACHMENT BONDS AND HEALING

What does the research tell us about adult connectedness and what constitutes a successful pair bond, the kind of bond that, at best, offers sanctuary and promotes healing?

The picture of distress in close relationships drawn by researchers such as John Gottman (1994) reveals the power of emotion and particular cycles of interaction to define the quality of love relationships. Distressed relationships are characterized by absorbing states of negative affect, and interactions in which partners blame, criticize, and withdraw from each other. A pattern of interaction in which one partner criticizes and becomes contemptuous while the other withdraws, shuts down, or stonewalls, is particularly predictive of divorce. The couple's facial expressions of emotion—for instance, the wife expressing contempt and the husband showing fear—also predict, with impressive accuracy, the future disruption of the relationship. Husbands who withdraw in situations of conflict and show no emotion are, in fact, likely to be highly physiologically aroused and to stay in this negative state longer than their wives. This is also true of the children who avoid a parent during a separation-reunion, as shown in infant attachment research. The conclusion of recent research on marital distress is that it is not the number of disagreements, or the expression of anger, or whether fights are resolved that makes the difference in defining a relationship; it is whether the couple can sustain emotional engagement (Gottman, 1994, 1999). This capacity involves being able to disrupt negative cycles of blame–withdraw—in which each partner pulls for negative responses from the other—and finding ways to reconnect. Happy, stable relationships are characterized by emotional engagement and responsiveness, whereby couples can step out of reactive aversiveness and soothe each other.

These conclusions fit very well with attachment theory. In all his writings, Bowlby stresses the emotional nature of the attachment bond and the power of emotion and emotional signals to organize interactions. It may be said that emotion is the "music of the attachment dance" (Johnson, 1996). Bowlby also stresses that emotional engagement is the crucial defining factor in close relationships. From the attachment perspective, negative cycles of blame/pursue and withdraw/distance are so harmful because they destroy the safety and responsiveness necessary for sustained emotional engagement and secure bonding. As attachment theory states, it is accessibility and responsiveness that count. Attachment theory offers a concise explanation for the patterns found in research on marital distress. Distressed partners tend to push for contact and responsiveness and, if necessary, become coercive to get a response. In attachment terms, any response is better than none. If there is no response from an attachment figure, there is no bond. What may be expected to resolve conflict and foster relationship satisfaction then is not so much new insights or new contracts about pragmatic issues, but the emotional attunement and responsiveness that make for a more secure bond.

The cycles of distress elaborated by the research on marital distress are best viewed as separation distress—specifically, as the protest and the seeking for contact that naturally accompany loss of emotional engagement and threats to attachment security. Such security needs naturally arise or become more intense at times of change, stress, and danger. How we frame distressed partners' responses will decide whether we see personality disorders, a situation calling for conflict management and negotiation skills, or a potentially adaptive struggle for the attachment security that promotes optimal adaptation. Distressed partners naturally speak of relationship distress in terms of attachment insecurity. For instance, in a couple session Mary says to her spouse, who is trying to rationally negotiate bedtime routines, "This is not about routines. You let me drown. I was drowning that night. So much had happened. And you turned out the light so you could be up for your important meeting the next day. When I needed you, you left me in the dark."

If relationship distress is seen in terms of attachment insecurity, it follows that when emotional engagement is urgently needed and is not achieved or is withheld, such events have a very significant impact on the definition of the relationship. As Simpson and Rholes (1994) have stated, the quality of a relationship is influenced out of all proportion by those occasions when one partner is seriously distressed and the other either responds and provides proximity or fails to do so. If the partner does respond, the bond is strengthened. If the partner does not respond at such times, these events then become traumatic stressors in themselves.

ATTACHMENT RELATIONSHIPS AND TRAUMA

The couple therapist is inevitably going to encounter couples whose relationship distress is preventing the development of the safe haven and secure base necessary for the healing of a specific trauma. In some cases a trauma, such as the loss of a child or a rape, negatively impacts a relationship, which was otherwise relatively secure, and provokes relationship distress. Consider the case of Clara. When she became ill with cancer and her husband coped with her situation by denial and emotional withdrawal, the relationship became distressed. This distress then began to undermine Clara's ability to deal with the traumatic crisis in her life. Her husband's response added to her sense of helplessness and was wounding in itself. The couple therapy process has to deal with this kind of attachment injury if such relationships are not only to improve, but also to provide platforms on which individual parties can stand and face the crises in their lives.

In many other cases, the situation is more complicated. For some veterans of war or victims of violence, or in cases of childhood sexual or physical abuse, when the trauma is of human design and often perpetrated by attachment figures, all close relationships tend to be contaminated by the trauma. The survivor as an individual and the couple as partners may never have known a safe attachment bond and may, in fact, have relatively rigid attachment styles that make the creation of such a bond difficult. In these cases, the lack of any kind of attachment security and the ongoing relationship distress seem to actively perpetuate the effects of trauma, and the effects of trauma perpetuate the relationship distress and the partners' insecure attachment styles. This becomes a self-reinforcing cycle that undermines other interventions, such as the survivor's individual therapy. The partner may also become vicariously traumatized. Both partners end up in absorbing states of insecurity and negative cycles of interaction that confirm the world and others as dangerous and themselves as helpless. Inner and outer patterns perpetuate themselves. There is no exit or respite. In this situation, trauma renders the need for safe attachment urgent and, at the same time, frames attachment relationships as direct sources of danger. The attachment figure becomes at once the source of, and the solution to, alarm. Both partners are caught in a paradox.

This process within a relationship seems to parallel the general symptoms of PTSD, in which hyperarousal, numbing, or both replace an integrated, organized response and paradoxically help to perpetuate the problem. In severely traumatized partners, a pattern of relating whereby individuals flip between hyperarousal and numbing parallels what child attachment theorists call a disorganized attachment style (Main & Hesse, 1990). In the language of adult attachment, this pattern constitutes what researchers term a fearful avoidant attachment style. Classically, this form of engagement, a further differentiation of avoidant attachment, involves needing closeness and pushing for it, but then, when it is offered, fearing and avoiding it and habitually viewing others as untrustworthy and the self as unlovable (Bartholomew & Horowitz, 1991). As a client, Carole, put it, "I need to know he is there and I get so angry when he isn't. I test him, I suppose. But then when he comes closer, I can't bear to be touched, so I space out and withdraw."

Those who have developed such an insecure style of engagement with others will find it harder to create relationships that offer a safe haven. They will be more susceptible to present stresses and traumatic events and less able to heal from past traumas. There is nothing so practical as a good theory. It is useful for the couple therapist to know the shapes insecurity take and how it may hamper the creation of trust and the creation of healing relationships (Johnson & Whiffen, 1999). Such insecurity impacts three core elements in relationship definition—affect regulation, information processing, and the process of communication between partners—as discussed in the following paragraphs.

Attachment and Affect Regulation and Expression

Attachment is a behavioral control system designed to promote physical proximity and achieve the emotional goal of "felt security" when individuals are threatened, vulnerable, or distressed. Proximity to a caregiver is an innate affect regulation device that soothes the nervous system. There is now evidence that the physical development of the neural structures that govern emotion are affected by attachment processes, such as emotional attunement between child and attachment figures (Schore, 1994). If a child or adult experiences fear, but has confidence that another will be present and responsive, there will be an expectation of relief and support. Fear, and the need to escape and protect the self, is then not so overwhelming, and fear cues will be dealt with effectively. If distress is created by the attachment relationship itself, the securely attached person has experienced interactive repair, and, again, distress is more manageable. Individuals with different attachment styles experience and deal with emotions differently. Securely attached people tend to openly acknowledge distress and turn to others for support in a way that elicits responsiveness.

Anxious, preoccupied partners are always afraid of losing attachment figures, so they tend to be reactive to affective cues and to amplify negative emotions by attending to them excessively. These individuals become easily anxious and angry, become absorbed in these emotions, and express them in an exaggerated manner. This style tends to drive others away, confirming all the anxious partner's fears.

In those with avoidant styles the awareness and expression of emotion, both positive and negative, are blunted and masked. The emotion is not neutralized, however; arousal is still high. The evidence is that emotional suppression is hard work and does not offer an escape from emotional pain (Gross & Levenson, 1993). In these individuals, emotion is expressed in somatization, hostility, and avoidance such as through obsession with instrumental tasks (Dozier & Kobak, 1992; Mikulincer et al., 1993). Emotion is inhibited, so it is not used as a source of information about needs and desires. Thus, a withdrawn-avoidant husband says to his partner, "I don't know what you mean. I have no idea what I need in this relationship. I just spend my time avoiding your anger and working on the computer where I can get tasks done and feel good about myself." Emotion is then not expressed at key moments in ways that send clear signals to a partner. Avoidant individuals avoid emotional engagement precisely at the moment when they or their partners experience vulnerability and need (Simpson et al., 1992), often leaving their partners feeling abandoned and rejected. A sense of security with a loved one facilitates engagement with and the effective processing of emotional responses. It also allows emotions to be expressed so as to clarify a person's goals and needs and foster supportive connections to others.

Attachment and Information Processing

Attachment styles involve more than the content of working models, expectations, and strategies. They also involve rules for processing and organizing information about the self, the world, and relationships. The primary purpose of working models is to enable a person to make predictions in attachment relationships (Shaver, Collins, & Clarke, 1996). Insecure models predispose people to selectively attend to and defensively distort information. The partner's behavior is usually interpreted in the interests of safety. This is, of course, even more pronounced in the case of trauma survivors who have been abused in close relationships. These clients are subject to suddenly being transported into past traumatic situations that are evoked by simple, everyday cues such as the touch of a partner's hand. Events occurring in the present that are inconsistent with existing models have the potential to modify a survivor's sense of the danger that accompanies closeness, but they require more attention and processing. This may be particularly difficult with a trauma survivor whose attention is split between being engaged in the present and, as one client put it "always having one eye on the dragon." As experts on emotion suggest, intense fear exercises such tight control over information processing that it typically eliminates all parts of the perceptual field that do not offer an escape route (Izard & Youngstrom, 1996). Intense, chronic fear reduces working memory, increases superficial processing of information, generates extensive cognitive bias, and preempts all other processing. Thus, when the therapist invites Julie to raise her head and look at her partner, who is openly reaching for her and offering to support and comfort her, she cannot. She is swamped with images of her father offering comfort and abusing her at the same time. She is certain that if she raises her head, she will see in Larry's eyes the disgust she feels for herself when these images arise. She needs considerable support from the therapist to see and emotionally connect with Larry's offer of caring.

Secure working models seem to promote cognitive exploration and flexibility (Main, 1991). Such exploration reflects the long-observed fact that children who trust the bond with their attachment figures go off and explore their universe more than children who do not. Individuals with a secure style are more open to new evidence (Mikulincer, 1997). They are more likely to rely on new information when making social judgments, are more curious, and can tolerate and deal with ambiguity better than insecure individuals. In contrast, insecure individuals respond more negatively to uncertainty and have a high need for closure. Avoidant persons especially tend to dismiss the significance of new information and to lack curiosity. In general, a secure style seems to facilitate learning from new experience. Secure partners are better able to consider alternative perspectives and see such perspectives as relative constructions rather than absolute realities. They are then better able to engage in collaborative problem solving. In interactions with partners, secure individuals seem less likely to jump to negative conclusions in the face of ambiguous signals and are better able to integrate new information into their view of their spouse.

There is also evidence that more secure people are better able to engage in meta-monitoring (Kobak & Cole, 1991; Main, Kaplan, & Cassidy, 1985). Meta-monitoring refers to the ability to step outside the action loop of goal-directed activity, form a coherent view of a relationship, and evaluate alternative strategies and perspectives. This ability parallels the ability to disengage from negative interactional cycles and initiate a more positive kind of interaction, which research on predictors of relationship distress identifies as crucial to the health of a relationship. Securely attached partners can remain constructive in response to their partners' potentially destructive behaviors (Rusbault, Verette, Whitney, Slovik, & Lipkus, 1991). They seem to be able to meta-monitor a conversation and to acknowledge and address communication difficulties in such a way that they become sources of new information and understanding (Kobak & Duemmler, 1994). They can focus on process as well as content. The ability to tolerate doubt and uncertainty, which can be fostered by a positive therapeutic alliance, is a prerequisite for the coordination of the emotional and attentional processes involved in meta-monitoring. More securely attached partners may then be expected to find it easier to grasp the nature of the negative cycles of interaction in their relationships and to frame these cycles, rather than the other spouse, as the enemy. This did seem to be the case in the research on couple therapy that my colleagues and I have conducted.

In addition, research that measures attachment by interviewing adults about their memories of attachment with their own parents suggests that secure individuals are able to take a meta-perspective in relationships. They are able to access, reflect on, and discuss attachment relationships and models in a coherent, integrated way (Main et al., 1985). Insecure individuals seem to have difficulty recalling and discussing their past attachment relationships. Avoidant individuals cannot recall, or give general idealized images that do not fit with, specific painful memories, and anxious, preoccupied individuals recall many specific incidents and conflicts, but cannot articulate a coherent overall picture of their attachment relationships. Formulating a coherent overview of a relationship that allows for the revision of perceptions and expectations logically seems to be a central task in recovering from negative experiences in past or ongoing relationships. This task will be more difficult for avoidant and preoccupied partners. *It is difficult to revise what one cannot access, coherently articulate, and evaluate.* In general, attachment insecurity involves a closed diversionary or closed hypervigilant style of information processing (Kobak & Cole, 1991). Insecurity acts to constrict and narrow the ways in which cognitions and affect are processed and thus to constrain key behavioral responses.

The ongoing process of making meaning of and learning about a relationship will be highly influenced by safety in those relationships. For survivors, meaning making is conducted with their toes over an emotional cliff.

Attachment and Communication Behaviors

A secure relationship seems to go hand in hand with emotionally open, fluent, and coherent communication, both within the attachment relationship and about the attachment relationship. Emotional communication is the link between partners' inner working models and the quality of their relationship (Bowlby, 1988; Kobak & Hazan, 1991). Secure partners find it easier to engage in open, direct, and coherent communication and give clear signals that help their partners to respond appropriately. In sum, a sense of felt security fosters communication competence (Anders & Tucker, 2000). In the relationships of insecure partners, absorbing states of negative affect prime forms of avoidant flight or anxious fight behavior. Consider June, who says to her anxiously attached husband, "But you don't ask me for help! You get real mad and tense and then say something really critical. And I'm so busy ducking, I can't even hear anything after that." Fight and flight behaviors then distort attachment signals and make positive emotional engagement in dialogue more difficult. An individual's habitual style of engagement and the working models implicit in that style will impact key communication behaviors, such as self-disclosure, empathic listening, assertiveness, and collaborative problem solving.

Trusting self-disclosure and empathic responsiveness are the basic building blocks of intimacy in relationships (Wynne & Wynne, 1986). Securely attached people disclose more and tend to be more responsive to their partners' self-disclosure, so it is easier for them to foster intimacy. In the simplest terms, such people are usually less focused on managing their own emotions and so find it easier to focus on and respond to those of others. As Goleman (1995, p. 112) suggests, "Attunement to others demands a modicum of calm in oneself." In contrast, avoidantly attached people are relatively unwilling to self-disclose and are not usually responsive to their partners self-disclosure. Anxious, preoccupied partners disclose, but often with compulsion and with an insensitivity to the other's needs. In terms of empathy, anxious and pre-occupied partners find it hard to focus on anything but their own emotions and attachment needs and so have difficulty seeing things from their partners' perspective. Avoidant partners' disengagement also makes it difficult for them to attune to others. In contrast, the secure person's confidence in the other's responsiveness fosters empathy and perspective taking (Mikulincer & Nachshon, 1991). Thus, a husband with a history of positive attachment relationships is able to tell his wife, "It's true, I would like more contact and more sexuality in our re-lationship, and it's hard not to take your distance as rejection. But I un-derstand that while you are dealing with the pain resulting from the rape, you need space and time to heal. I just want you to know that I am here and want to help you feel safe."

In situations of conflict, security is associated with balanced asser-tiveness (Kobak & Sceery, 1988). Secure partners offer more support and use rejection less, whereas anxious attachment is linked to dysfunc-tional anger and the use of coercion. Security is related to a lack of ver-bal aggression during problem solving and to a lack of withdrawal (Senchak & Leonard, 1992). Research thus suggests that attachment se-curity enhances the ability to communicate openly, to negotiate, and to collaborate in problem solving (Kobak & Hazan, 1991). Communica-tion behaviors are context dependent; when stress is low, avoidantly at-tached persons may engage in open conversation. However, the quality of an attachment relationship tends to be defined by those moments when risks are taken and vulnerabilities shared and responded to. At such moments, a couple's ability to disclose and confide clearly and directly about their needs and fears, to respond to each other empath-ically, and to consider alternatives is crucial if they are to experience the relationship as a secure base.

On a more general note, attachment theory assumes that we are all children of the same mother. Attachment needs and processes are as-sumed to be universal and to be reflected in all cultures. However, as stated previously, research has also found differences across cultures, particularly in terms of perspectives and in display rules between indi-vidual-oriented cultures, such as North America, and collectivistic cul-tures, such as Japan (Rothbaum et al., 2000). It is important that the therapist learn about and respect both partners' cultural backgrounds as they relate to attachment relationships and to modes of coping with traumatic experiences. Models of therapy that focus on how individuals continually construct their experiences and their interactions with others may be better able to respond to and take cultural differences into account. There are often as many differences between individuals within a culture as there are between cultures. For example, it may be quite difficult for a couple therapist who has no familiarity with the military to connect with war veterans. Although, as one veteran told me, "It's okay—I get this bonding stuff. In the marines you had to be tough, but the motto was, a marine never leaves another marine. You don't fight a war alone, you know. It's when you come home that you feel alone."

ATTACHMENT STYLES AND TRAUMA SURVIVORS

Many trauma survivors who seek therapy struggle with the problems of insecure attachment discussed earlier. These problems are made more intense and are infinitely compounded by trauma symptoms. The aftereffects of trauma ensure that survivors will have even greater difficulty with affect regulation, for example, than distressed, insecure partners who have never faced trauma. Trauma survivors are often trying to fight two battles at the same time. They are fighting the cycles of distress in their relationships and are also fighting the echoes of traumatic events that are evoked constantly by that relationship. It makes sense that these individuals experience more trouble with affect regulation, information processing, and interpersonal communication. It is also a tribute to the strength of the human spirit and the power of attachment needs that they are willing to wrestle with their fears to connect with the ones they love.

The sources of soothing and islands of comfort and hope that many distressed couples are still able to find in their relationships are often not available to traumatized couples. A stable relationship seems to require that there is more than double the amount of positive than negative feeling expressed (Gottman, 1994). Maintaining this proportion may be a tall order for trauma survivors. A survivor also needs more support from a spouse and yet is less able to ask for it. The spouse is often confused and overwhelmed and may not even know the exact nature of the trauma his or her partner is facing.

Research into adult attachment styles has recently differentiated the avoidant style into two types: dismissing avoidance, in which attachment needs are denied, and fearful avoidance, in which individuals desire contact with others but are also very withdrawn and afraid of such contact. The behavior of fearful-avoidant partners is often a chaotic mix of avoidance and seeking and clinging. We know that survivors, particularly of CSA, who often suffer from complex PTSD, are much more likely than most to have fearful-avoidant attachment styles (Shaver & Clarke, 1994). The ambivalent and contradictory interactional style of many of these adult survivors of abuse can be captured in the image of an abused or neglected child whose mother comes into a room after a separation. The child runs toward the mother, anxious for contact. But just before she reaches her mother, the child stops. She is suddenly flooded with fear about the dangers inherent in this contact, and so she turns her back to her mother and walks toward her backward. This behavior appears bizarre, but as suggested earlier, the child (like fearful-avoidant partners) is in a paradoxical situation in which contact is both a source of and a solution to terror and her behavior is, in fact, a perfectly rational attempt to deal with her opposing needs and fears. One study found that 58% of women who were incestuously abused were fearful-avoidant in their attachments, and those who did not fall into this group tended to demonstrate an anxious attachment style. These two styles, anxious and fearful-avoidant, are those associated with a negative model of self; however, fearful-avoidant women tend to have the most negative self-concepts, viewing themselves as helpless and hopeless. They are also most likely to be depressed. In fact, on every measure of mental health these women are found to be the worst off (Alexander, 1993; Shaver & Clarke, 1994).

In our hospital clinic, we found that such women (and male survivors of CSA as well) viewed their bodies as an enemy and often engaged in self-mutilation and self-destructive behavior. It has been suggested that this fearful-avoidant style may be generally the most difficult style to update and modify in new relationship contexts, although in a preliminary couple therapy study we did find we could foster changes in model of self in these partners, at least in the short term (Sims, 1999). These survivors have particular problems in being able to stand back and gain some perspective on their relationships (Main et al., 1985). As stated before, it is hard to revise what you cannot access, clarify, and evaluate. Complex PTSD, which characterizes CSA survivors (Herman, 1993), may be what naturally occurs when there is only the dragon and the dark. It is the result of facing prolonged and repeated trauma without a safe haven or connection with caring others. In such isolation, human beings and other primates have to develop desperate survival tactics such as dissociating—in essence, not being there—or self-injury. Primate research has amply demonstrated that self-mutilation is a common reaction to social isolation and inescapable fear (Suomi, 1989). *Isolation from others becomes as pernicious in its effects as traumatic abuse itself.* Ways of coping, such as dissociation, make revictimization more likely and tend to perpetuate insecurity and relationship difficulties. The experience of my colleagues and I has been that once we understood the paradox inherent in their experience of attachment and were able to deal with the confusing, fluid emotional states of fearful-avoidant survivors, they did respond to couple therapy interventions, perhaps because part of them still longed for closeness. The clients, traumatized or not, whom we find most difficult to reach are partners who use extreme avoidant-dismissing strategies and who also rigidly hold onto their models of self and other. These partners are also less likely to agree to engage in couple therapy.

There is yet another issue for these survivors. McCann and Pearlman (1990) emphasize that apart from the ability to manage affect and connect with others, the capacity most affected by trauma such as CSA is the ability to maintain a positive sense of self. In terms of attachment style, both anxious and fearful-avoidant individuals tend to have a negative model of self, whereas dismissing-avoidant and secure individuals express more confidence about their self-worth. Fearful individuals particularly tend to be introverted and to lack social self-confidence. If we look more closely, this issue breaks down into the following points :

- These survivors tend to have a more fragile sense of self; it is less coherent and integrated. The process of self-construal is disorganized.
- Their sense of self is not simply negative, it is usually flooded with acute shame and self-disgust. They actively blame themselves for what has happened to them. Such self-blame has often been actively fostered by the perpetrator. The content of the schemas defining the self is thus extremely negative.
- The self is actively mistrusted and despised. Bowlby (1988) states that a key feature in the development of working models of self is how acceptable or unacceptable a person is in the eyes of attachment figures. Many survivors have never experienced an affirming and accepting attachment figure to mirror a lovable sense of self. Thus, it is not surprising when a survivor comments to a couple therapist, "To be honest, I've never known why he is still

with me. I am just such a disgusting mess inside. I can't imagine why anyone would ever want me."

How might we understand these survivors' fragile sense of self from an attachment perspective? First, constructing a coherent sense of self is very difficult for a child engaged in what attachment theorists call a disorganized, disorienting relationship. The child depends not only on the physical contact of the parent for security, but also on the mind of the parent to help the child structure experience and mirror a predictable coherent sense of self. For clients such as Charlene, discussed in Chapter 6, whose mother was dying of cancer all through her childhood and who was parented by an exceedingly hostile cousin whose sons violently sexually abused her, it is natural to experience themselves in conflicting fragments. In her counseling sessions Charlene would alternate between experiencing herself as a toxic child who does not deserve love, as an enraged adult who knows that she was victimized and needs comfort from her distant spouse, and then as a "numb" mother who feels that she has to stay distant from her own children to avoid hurting them. In the same breath, Charlene would talk of her hurt as an abandoned child and of her contempt for herself as a "poor little sucky orphan," as her cousin used to label her.

It is also useful to remember that working models, as delineated by Bowlby (1969), are interpersonal and relational. Self-concept is always in relation to others. The potentially available images used to construct a sense of self are formed and stored in the context of self-and-other interactions. A predictable, consistent parent also teaches a child to link inner emotion to behavioral response in a consistent way, and to process experience and act in congruent way. This parent then helps the child construct a coherent sense of self. However, coping with an abusive parent most often requires the denial of feelings and needs and a break between impulse and act, thought and speech.

There is also research on how people with different styles organize their self-concepts. Various aspects of adult attachment have been measured in different ways: first, by self-report questionnaires that focus on inner thoughts and feelings about self and others, and second, by interviews, such as Main's Adult Attachment Interview (AAI; George, Kaplan, & Main, 1984). This interview assesses observable defenses and how people think of and talk about attachment relationships, mostly past relationships with parents, in the present. In a recent research project, pregnant mothers were interviewed on the AAI. Among the conclusions of this project was that those with secure attachment styles are free to evaluate attachment experiences. These mothers showed a coherence of discourse, which seemed to reflect a coherence of mind about attachment issues. If they spoke in a coherent, integrated way about their past and present attachment experiences (even if those experiences were negative or even abusive in the past), these mothers tended to have children who at 18 months showed secure responses in staged separations. A child's behavior in such separations can be predicted with 80% accuracy from the parent's responses on the AAI (Fonagy, Steele, & Steele, 1991). If the mother was able to reflect on ideas related to attachment in an integrated way (such as recognizing different ways of interpreting her own mother's or her child's responses to her and acknowledging that her attachment figures had their own problems and defenses), her child demonstrated secure behavioral responses in a stressful situation. It seems likely that accurate, coherent communication on the part of the mother regarding attachment-related emotions is the major determinant of a child's later attachment style (Shaver et al., 1996). A mother who is able to stand back, reflect on attachment, and talk about attachment-related feelings models for her child a theory of mind. She helps her child detect and act on feelings in a coherent way. The child then "finds himself in the other." Researchers such as Fonagy (Fonagy et al., 1995) believe that just one secure attachment relationship is enough to teach this ability to reflect on the inner states of the self and the other. They also believe that this protects people from the most pernicious effects of trauma, such as the development of personality disorders with their fragmented sense of self.

In addition, survival mechanisms such as dissociation and numbing naturally lead to discontinuous experience of self. Survivors constantly doubt their own perceptions and need the affirmation of supportive others. The sense of self is evoked very powerfully in interactions with partners that focus on attachment issues (see the session transcript in Johnson & Williams Keeler, 1998). The couple therapist must constantly be aware of survivors' sensitivity to this element of the interaction.

COUPLE THERAPY WITH TRAUMATIZED CLIENTS

What would a couple therapist hope for in the best of all possible outcomes with a traumatized couple? The therapist would hope that the partners would be able to offer each other comfort and reassuring support. More specifically, the partners would:

- Experience not only general insight into their problems or an increase in positive factors such as ease of communication, but also a sense of safe emotional connectedness. The ability to soothe and comfort and respond to vulnerability is crucial from an attachment perspective. In research on predictors of marital distress (Gottman et al., 1998), this aspect of relationships is also now identified as crucial to relationship satisfaction.
- Respond to each other in a way that not only allows them to step out of reactive cycles of distress but also allows them to stand together at times when intrusive symptoms such as flashbacks or nightmares occur. When the partner becomes an ally in regulating a survivor's feelings of helplessness, more problematic ways of fending off such helplessness can be short-circuited.
- Confide in each other about the impact the trauma has had on both their lives. As the relationship becomes a more secure base, numbing begins to lessen. Secrecy and inhibition are often the rule in traumatized couples' relationships. Confiding not only builds trust with the partner, it also encourages the processing and reorganization of the experience that is confided.
- Use the relationship as a source of comfort to deal with hyperarousal and irritation, and differentiate trauma triggers so that the partner can offer support rather than be a bystander or even a target.
- Reach for and comfort each other when attachment needs arise, and with them grief, fear of abandonment, and helplessness. A corrective experience can then occur that is incompatible with the violation that was often part of the trauma experience for the survivor. Partners have often been vicariously traumatized, and they too need comfort and reassurance.
- Offer acceptance and reassurance to each other, which challenge models of self as unworthy and deserving of the hurt that has been inflicted. To be seen and understood by the one we love best may be the most powerful weapon against shame.
- Share a common worldview about the meaning of the trauma, the state of mind of the perpetrator, and the survivor's state of mind during and after the trauma. It is never too late to construct

a coherent, meaningful account of a trauma and the identity of
the person who experienced it.

- Strategize about how to protect their present relationship and
each other in case of future incursions of trauma.
- Actively use, by the end of couple therapy, the best in-wired antidote we have against debilitating fear, the comfort of each other.

To help a traumatized couple, a therapist must have a clear map of
close relationships and how aspects of such relationships help or hinder
facing the dragon of trauma. The therapist also needs techniques for
dealing with emotion and using it to create new kinds of interactions.
Specifically, the therapist must help partners de-escalate the negative cycles that feed the dragon, and foster the emotional engagement and responsiveness that promote healing from the dragon's fire.

In the following chapters, the interventions and examples are de-
rived from emotionally focused couple therapy (EFT). This models fits
well for trauma survivors, based as it is on an attachment perspective
and offering a focus on emotion and emotional engagement. In constructivist information-processing terms, emotion is seen here as an integration of physiological responses to survival-related cues and meaning schemes, and as a set of action tendencies (for example, fear evokes
flight or withdrawal), as well as the self-reflexive awareness of this experience and a set of strategies to manage it (Johnson, 1996). EFT has
been used with different kinds of trauma survivors (Johnson, in press;
Johnson & Williams Keeler, 1998). The implementation of EFT with
distressed partners displaying different kinds of attachment styles has
also been outlined (Johnson & Whiffen, 1999). Furthermore, there is
literature and research applying EFT to clinical depression, which frequently accompanies PTSD (Johnson et al., 1999; Whiffen & Johnson,
1998). A number of relevant interventions taken from other models of
couple therapy are referred to briefly.

Given the incidence of trauma, it is inevitable that all couple therapists, sooner or later, find themselves dealing with traumatized couples.
Any therapist who hopes to help such couples must be both active and
nonpathologizing in his or her approach, and the interventions referred
to here reflect these requirements.

Chapter 4

Assessment

When traumatized partners first engage in couple therapy, the therapist finds him- or herself dealing with a complex picture. The therapist has to come to an understanding of the impact of traumatic experience on both partners and the relationship, how this experience blocks relationship repair, and the nature of the general distress in the relationship. There are often other problems present as well. The most frequently encountered additional problem is depression in one or both partners. The complexity of this picture requires a "pragmatic, holistic and integrated theory" (Wilson & Kurtz, 1997, p. 350) that allows the therapist to bring all the elements into focus in an assessment. The assessment then becomes both a first step toward change and a guide to the change process.

As suggested in previous chapters, attachment theory provides the couple therapist with a map to intimate relationships. Beginning with the first session, this map allows the therapist to stay focused and out of the quicksand of dealing with every element of the trauma and its consequences. This chapter summarizes the key dimensions of the assessment process, suggests a few assessment instruments, and presents some of the key issues that arise in a first assessment interview.

Nearly all clients who seek a couple therapist are frustrated and in pain, but some are also carrying the weight of traumatic experience. The level of personal awareness, the integration of the traumatic experience, and the significance of the trauma for the relationship, as well as couple's ability to deal with this experience, will differ among couples. Some partners will have already confronted, perhaps even "tamed," their trauma, whether it is a recent, relatively contained event, such as a violent crime or rape or a fight with cancer, or a past complex trauma, such as childhood sexual abuse. These partners now want to address the specific impact of the trauma on their everyday interactions. Some partners, however, come to couple therapy before they have even named their personal trauma. The following are examples of the different ways the dragon is revealed in the couple therapist's office. Most of these synopses introduce couples whose stories are discussed at greater length in subsequent chapters.

1. *The dragon tamed and minimal relationship distress.* Referred by their concerned physician, Mary and Joe come to the clinic to talk about their relationship and the stress of having their 17-year-old son leave home. Joe, the husband, is asphasic. He has learned to speak again after the trauma of a stroke of 5 years ago, but we include his speech therapist in the session, write things on a pad for him to make sure he understands, and use the technique of reflection to help him express his message clearly. This couple are clear that Joe's stroke was exceedingly traumatic for both of them, but their story and the way they interact in the session show that they have dealt with this trauma very well. They appear to have been able to maintain a vibrant bond. They each speak openly and empathically of the other's bravery and how they "wept and held each other" throughout the crisis and during the long recovery and adjustment period. They tell of rituals of comfort and soothing that they have created in their relationship and the creative ways they have used to accommodate to Joe's disability, including finding him a new career. Facing the dragon together makes bonds stronger. During the session, they encapsulate their positions concerning their son and chat relatively amicably about their fears and concerns about his leaving home. With minimal help from the therapist, they work to solve problems and formulate an approach to dealing with their son. At the end of the assessment the couple and the therapist agree that they do not seem to need couple therapy at the moment. In fact, his speech therapist later reported that Joe went on to proudly tell his aphasia group that he was much more an expert on close relationships than he thought he was.

2. *The dragon in disguise and untamed and severe relationship distress.* Charlene and Jim come to the clinic complaining of relationship distress and describe how Charlene's severe eating disorder creates distance between them. As they talk, however, Charlene refers to a

childhood marked by loss and sexual abuse. She does not link these events to her responses in the relationship and does not even label them as traumatic. She has never been assessed or treated for posttraumatic stress disorder (PTSD). All therapeutic efforts have focused on the symptoms of her eating disorder, which have not changed over the last 2 years. To the therapist it is clear that Charlene's trauma is significant, untouched, and does indeed have an impact on the relationship both generally (she describes herself as either withdrawn or irritable) and in more specific ways (she cannot tolerate any sexual touch). In spite of the many serious problems this couple face, they both affirm their commitment to the relationship and their willingness to learn how to deal with their issues. This couple's journey through therapy is described in Chapter 6.

3. *The dragon barely held in check and severe relationship distress.* David and Joan come to couple therapy at the insistence of David's individual therapist, who sees him for problems with anxiety. David describes a horrendous childhood spent trying to protect himself from his very violent, abusive father. Both he and Joan are able to describe how the patterns he learned with his father have always interfered with their relationship. Now, after 35 years, Joan cannot deal with his anger and "need for control" and says she is leaving. David's trauma, which has been explicitly addressed in many sessions of individual therapy, is acknowledged by both partners as affecting the relationship in specific ways, particularly through David's need for control and his emotional abusiveness. In this couple, the trauma and its impact on the relationship have been identified, and David has addressed and reduced many of his intrusive symptoms. However, both partners feel overwhelmed and unable to deal with their distress. Joan also tells of a lonely childhood full of danger and despair. This couple's therapeutic process is described in Chapter 7.

4. *The dragon of current illness and severe relationship distress.* Len and Clara come to therapy because Clara has stated that she is leaving their marriage of 42 years. She is in individual therapy, and her therapist reports she is doing well and coping well with her relatively recent cancer diagnosis and illness. Her cancer is now in remission; however, her spouse has just retired and has become clinically depressed. As Clara describes it, her fight with cancer seems to have damaged the marriage irrevocably. The trauma here is recent and acknowledged and the survivor is coping; however, it has negatively impacted the relationship, which is now deeply distressed. There is also concern for the future, inasmuch as Clara's cancer will almost certainly recur, and she

says, "Since I am alone anyway, I would rather simply live alone." This couple's story is presented in Chapter 8.

5. *The dragon of war, almost tamed, and severe relationship distress.* Rob and Elizabeth come to therapy after Rob has been assessed for PTSD as a result of his two tours of duty in Vietnam. He has received some individual therapy over the years and has been in a veteran's therapy group. The trauma here is long term and has been addressed on an individual level, with some success, and in the group, but key relational issues have not been addressed and are now primary. One of the ways Rob has dealt with his memories has been by drinking, and his marriage has become exceedingly distressed over the last year. When his wife stated that she was going to leave him, he told her he would leave first, but then he might commit suicide. This couple is presented in Chapter 9.

6. *Relationship trauma and terminal relationship distress.* Mary and Chad come to the clinic because Mary has thrown separation papers in Chad's face and told him she is leaving him. Chad is a very traditional man who exemplifies an avoidant-dismissing attachment style, and has stated adamantly that he does not believe in therapy; however, he also does not want to be divorced. As the couple tells their story, Mary returns again and again to Chad's response to her first miscarriage, which, as she described it, was to coldly criticize her, suggest that her family were defective in terms of physical resilience, and keep his distance, no matter how upset she became. Although the couple begins to make some progress, Mary returns again and again to this event as epitomizing her experience of the relationship. After a few sessions, Chad announces that he is not willing to work on the relationship because Mary has, in fact, decided never to trust him again and is going to leave anyway. She then agrees that because their everyday interactions still reflect the pattern apparent in the miscarriage incident and she is becoming clearer about her own needs, she does not want to trust Chad again and wishes to separate. The pivotal relationship trauma described here defines this relationship as insecure and blocks its repair. Relationship traumas of this kind, and how the therapist can deal with them, are addressed in Chapter 10 in the case of Lou and John.

FIRST SESSIONS: KEY DIMENSIONS

Certain key dimensions emerge from just a cursory glance at the aforementioned cases:

• *Level of trauma.* Is the trauma a relatively contained one-time event, such as a car accident or an assault, occurring in the context of flexible coping skills? Or is the trauma one that is chronic and central in a partner's past relationships and an active factor in this partner's development and present construal of self and the other? The latter kind of trauma tends to evoke complex PTSD (Herman, 1993). Complex PTSD is characterized by a multiplicity of symptoms, diffuse problems in all facets of personality, including cognitive, behavioral, somatic, affective, and interpersonal, and a vulnerability to retraumatization.

• *Personal/relationship trauma.* Are the main signs of trauma specific to the relationship and tied to a specific incident that has undermined the security of the attachment bond in this particular relationship? In such cases, the other partner is the agent of the trauma. For example, the other partner has abandoned his or her spouse at a time of serious illness or crisis. From the perspective used in this text, these traumas can be termed attachment injuries and must be addressed in couple therapy if the relationship is to substantially improve and remain stable.

• *Level of personal integration of the trauma.* Does the survivor acknowledge the impact of the traumatic experience, and is this individual actively dealing with the impact of this experience? Does the trauma survivor presently have good coping strategies that limit the scope of the trauma's impact?

• *Level of integration of trauma into the relationship.* Has the nature of the trauma been shared with the nontraumatized partner? Do both partners understand how the trauma affects the way they "dance" together and dictates some of the specific steps in that dance? Have the couple found any coping strategies to deal positively with the impact of the trauma on their relationship? The majority of traumatized couples seeking couple therapy will be facing particular difficulties in integrating the effects of trauma into their relationship in a way that promotes secure bonding.

On a more general level, systemically oriented couple therapists tend to work within a brief time frame, and just as for real estate the key element is "location, location, location," the key feature for such therapy is "focus, focus, focus" (Donovan, 1999, p. 3). An important element of beginning sessions is the development of such a focus. Systemic therapists tend to concentrate on the present manner in which relationship problems maintain trauma symptoms. The extent to which, and manner in which, the therapist focuses on how trauma symptoms also maintain relationship problems (a more "internal" focus) may differ, depending on the therapist's orientation. Some therapists may focus just on specific behaviors related to the trauma, others may focus exclusively on cognitions. An EFT therapist follows a model that focuses on the way the system, the couple's interactions, is constructed and the way each partner also constructs his or her emotional experience of the relationship, paying particular attention to attachment needs and fears.

IS TRAUMA PART OF THE RELATIONSHIP PROBLEM?

Not all partners are able to disclose their traumatic experiences when they first meet with a couple therapist. What questions might such a therapist keep in mind when working with couples that would alert the therapist to the dragon lurking in the shadows of the relationship and help him or her understand the nature of this beast? A list of such questions may include the following:

- Is there any indication in the couple's story that some specific trauma has occurred that may play a part in the definition of this couple's relationship? If other professionals have referred the couple for therapy, do they mention traumatic experience as part of the picture?
- Do the partners mention, however briefly, that a particularly significant and overwhelming experience has occurred in their personal lives and/or relational life and that this experience still affects their life, even if specific links to present problems are not clear.
- Does the couple's problem cycle contain responses that in nature and intensity seem to resemble PTSD, or do partners discuss specific areas, such as intimate touch, with obvious distaste or shame?
- Do the partners show particular responses in the session, such as signs of dissociation, that suggest that a partner is facing overwhelming emotions that elicit extreme fight, flight, or flee methods of coping?
- Does either of the partners demonstrate a fearful-avoidant attachment style that manifests as extreme neediness and extreme

distrust and ambivalence about closeness with the partner, the therapist, or both? Such a style most often develops as part of the aftermath of trauma.

PTSD symptoms tend to create the same kinds of couple problems as extreme cycles of relationship distress. Constricted intimacy and expressiveness, overt hostility, and general problems in adjustment and depression (Caroll, Foy, Cannon, & Zwler, 1991; Silver & Iacono, 1986) are symptoms of PTSD and often part of the disintegration of a distressed relationship. However, the marks of the dragon are not usually very difficult to see.

TREATMENT VIABILITY

One of the tasks of the first few sessions is to evaluate whether intervention is presently viable. There are obvious difficulties that preclude the use of couple therapy, such as ongoing violence, uncontrolled drug abuse, or a couple's incompatible goals. For example, one person may have already left the relationship and may wish to stay separate, whereas the other wishes to renew the relationship. However, it is useful to consider treatment viability in more general terms. As Gurman (2001) points out, clients who present themselves as rigid and consistently externalize their difficulties, insist on keeping secrets that are relationally significant, and do not express commitment to a relationship are unlikely to take an active role in the change process. They are probably best thought of as "precontemplative," according to Prochaska's Stages of Change Model (Prochaska, Norcross, & DiClemente, 1994), and often leave therapy after a few sessions, no matter how empathic the therapist or how appropriate the model of therapy used.

Part of setting the framework for treatment is a discussion of treatment goals. Specifically, it is important to ask what each partner wants the relationship to look like at the end of a "successful" intervention. For treatment to be viable, there must be some compatibility between such goals. However, with traumatized couples it may be impossible for survivors to conceptualize or articulate an image of a trusting, close relationship. They may not know what such a relationship looks like. Such clients are also likely to be ambivalent and unsure as to how much closeness and trust they are interested in creating. The therapist may then have to help these clients construct an image of a preferred relationship that would address their present concerns, while leaving room for treatment goals to become more specific and concrete as treatment evolves. A theory of close relationships such as attachment theory offers the therapist a map to people's longings and needs. The therapist can then more easily tune into such needs and bring them from the background to center stage. For couples in whom the trauma is untouched, the goal of couples treatment may be the stabilization of the relationship so that it can provide a secure base, a platform for the survivor to begin to touch and come to terms with the traumatic experience. The EFT therapist would term this process de-escalation. Such a couple may then return to couple therapy at a later date to further increase the intimacy of their bond. Other couples, who have moved toward taming their dragon, can and do commit to clear goals, especially if the therapist can help them to define their dance and the part the dragon plays in it.

SAFETY NETS

From the beginning, the therapist who deals with a traumatized couple needs to erect safety nets. The therapist needs to ask explicitly, in individual and conjoint sessions, about whether any negative or harmful ways of dealing with trauma symptoms have been used, such as self-mutilation or drug abuse, and then explore ways to contain these toxic coping strategies.

An exploration of issues of violence and substance abuse is a crucial part of the construction of a safety net. If such issues are significant, they often preclude the implementation of couple therapy. Even if such an issue is not a factor in the present relationship, it may be important to discuss it, particularly if it has arisen in the past. Thus, a survivor who sought individual therapy because she was becoming abusive with her children was asked to stipulate times of particular stress when she found parenting difficult. She was then helped to specify how she might neutralize such incidents if they occurred again. These issues are discussed in the upcoming chapter on interventions.

Another safety net is created by actively posing potential anxiety-creating situations that may arise in the process of therapy, such as confiding the specific nature of the trauma to one's spouse for the first time, and structuring with the client specific ways of handling such situations. This is an ongoing process, because partners sometimes find it

hard to deal with such problems more positively until they have first begun to redefine their relationship. Consulting with other therapists involved is obviously helpful here. It is important to ask whether the client has a history of suicidal gestures or any kind of coping that can be
seen as self-harm. If so, does this person have a contract with his or her
individual therapist about what to do when thoughts of these actions
become compelling? If there is no such contract, it is advisable to create
one with this person as to what he or she can do if the change process
or, more specifically, the couple sessions, become overwhelming at any
point. For example, the couple therapist can stipulate regular times
when clients can contact him or her and offer a number of alternatives
they can turn to if they cannot contact the couple therapist or the survivor's individual therapist.

It is also useful to establish a predictable process whereby at the
end of each session the therapist asks about how each partner experienced the session, whether he or she needs any additional support for
the upcoming week, and what this support might ideally be. A usual
pattern is that initial sessions, and then later sessions in which partners,
especially the survivor, are beginning to take risks and move into new
kinds of dialogues and dances, are potentially the most overwhelming.
As part of the safety net, the therapist should actively encourage partners to state limits or concerns during the process of therapy, and give
assurances that such limits will be respected. Thus, at the beginning of
therapy, the therapist might state, "If at any time I ask you to touch or
talk about something too difficult, or confide in your partner in a way
that feels too overwhelming for you, I want you to tell me, and we will
slow things down and respect your feelings."

The best safety net of all is a positive therapeutic alliance.

THE THERAPEUTIC ALLIANCE

The therapeutic alliance can be considered within the framework suggested by Gurman and Lebow (2000), which views the therapist as
adopting three possible roles: coach/educator, perturbator, or healer.
The couple therapist can be all three at various times, but in the context
of this book is most appropriately viewed as a healer. The therapist does
educate the couple—about the nature of trauma, for example, and the
nature of secure attachment. The therapist does stir up the system, for
example, by asking partners to state their unspoken fears and resent-

ments or to make explicit the positions they take in the relationship. For instance, a therapist may encourage a wife to engage her husband directly and say what has been unspoken, such as, "One part of me never wants to let you in—says it will never trust you." However, the therapist ultimately relies on creating a secure and responsive connection with distressed partners that offers them the safety to take new risks and create a corrective emotionally healing experience.

The connection with the therapist is an active part of the healing process, especially for partners whose connections with others have been so fraught with pain and uncertainty. Thus, a crucial aspect of early sessions is the process whereby the therapist not only listens to and helps partners to organize the story of their relationship, but also empathically attunes to each partner's position in the relational dance. Empathy is a leap of imagination (Guerney, 1994). The therapist engages in each client's experience in a way that clarifies this experience for the particular client. The therapist must be willing to be confused, lost, and unsure. He or she must be willing to go to the leading edge of the client's experience with the client and struggle to grasp and make sense of that experience. To do this, a certain acceptance of the partners and their vagaries is essential. A judgmental stance interferes with empathic attunement and naturally produces wariness and inhibition in clients. Moreover, the honoring of clients and their experiences models for them a compassionate, caring attitude toward each other.

A genuine relationship between therapist and client implies that the therapist allows him- or herself to be seen. The more predictable and visible the therapist is, the easier it will be for a trauma survivor and his or her partner to begin to trust that therapist. Therefore, it is important, in early sessions, for the therapist to respond in a genuine, congruent way to the couple's questions or challenges. Part of the excitement and the deep satisfaction in working with traumatized couples is that each couple teaches the therapist something new about people's resourcefulness in struggling with the dilemmas of being human and staying connected to others. For the therapist, working with such couples, who live more poignantly at the existential edge, can and perhaps should constitute an expansion of self (Arons & Arons, 1997). This implies that the therapist engages with each partner in a genuine, relatively open relationship.

Another way to conceptualize the therapeutic alliance is in terms of attachment. Positive attachments are characterized by accessibility and responsiveness. The therapist is not an attachment figure per se, and accessibility is obviously limited. However, to be as accessible and responsive as possible, while remaining within the confines of the role of therapist, seems to be a positive model. It involves the therapist's being aware of and honoring, when possible, the bids clients make for particular responses from him or her, bids for respect, acknowledgment, or comfort. Clients may need to know, for example, that the therapist is also willing to learn from them and that the therapist can make mistakes, such as underestimating how difficult a new step is for them, or how scorching the dragon's fire can be.

In particular, the therapist is a provider of structure and, when necessary, comfort. As traumatized clients tell their stories, they may become increasingly excited, angry, or tangential and disorganized, particularly if they have not addressed their issues in individual therapy. It is important that the therapist then provide structure to calm and stabilize such clients. Reflecting the reality the client is trying to express and helping the client to organize this reality into a coherent whole is often calming in itself. Emotions, when placed in context, become less overwhelming, and, in fact, act as guides to the meanings of events and the needs implicit in them. An actively validating stance toward each partner also provides reassurance. This involves not just nonpathologizing, but explicitly framing survival as success, negative behaviors as creative adaptations to impossible circumstances, and willingness to continue to confront the dragon as bravery and strength.

The alliance can also be framed in terms of the bond between therapist and clients, as referred to earlier, an agreement as to the goals of therapy, and the presentation of tasks that are relevant and generative for clients. The goals for traumatized clients coming to couple therapy may differ according to the level of integration of the trauma. As previously described, some clients may need to stabilize their relationship before engaging in the task of confronting a trauma on a personal level. Other clients, who have already confronted the trauma and begun to integrate it on a personal level, want to create a new bond that is less constrained by the insecurities that the trauma induced. Still other clients are dealing with relationship distress compounded by a relationship trauma that has to be resolved. Thus, the active negotiation of goals is part of early therapy sessions. *The relevance of the tasks set by the therapist should be transparent; that is, the therapist should be explicit and more than willing to discuss at any time what he or she is doing and why. The therapist should invite regular feedback from both partners about how they experience the therapy process.* A focus on emotion and attachment issues also helps to ensure that clients find the tasks set for them in therapy to be relevant and "on target." The perceived relevance of the tasks set by the therapist is the aspect of the therapeutic alliance that best predicts success in EFT (Johnson & Talitman, 1997).

In general, in EFT, as well as in the more dynamic therapies and the explicitly postmodern therapies such as narrative therapy, the main assessment "tool" includes the observation of how clients engage with the therapist and partners, the compilation of client's "stories" of their experiences, and attention to how they understand their problems. Therapeutic directions and goals are then constructed with the clients. There are, however, a number of more formal assessment tools. These tools, or instruments, can be useful adjuncts to the aforementioned process. They can, at times, make the assessment process more efficient or offer a way into the process itself.

ASSESSMENT INSTRUMENTS

Completing measures such as the Dyadic Adjustment Scale (Busby, Christensen, Crane, & Larson, 1995; Spanier, 1976) can give the therapist a quick sense of how a couple see their relationship relative to those of other distressed couples. This scale consists of 32 questions concerning overall happiness, satisfaction and commitment, consensus on various issues, and perceived levels of cohesion. On this measure, a score of 70 is typical of divorcing couples and 100 is the usual cutoff point for designating relationship distress used in research studies. Couples who score above this point after treatment are considered to have recovered from such distress.

The Relationship Trust Scale (Holmes, Boon, & Adams, 1990) can also be useful. The subscales in this 30-item test, Responsiveness, Reliability, Faith in Partner's Caring, Conflict Efficacy, and Dependency Concerns, have been revised to make it compatible with empirical findings regarding issues of insecurity in marriage and attachment styles, and the measure has good statistical reliability. In particular, it can help reticent partners begin to talk about attachment issues in their relationship, as well as give the therapist an overall sense of how the partners experience these particular issues.

A measure of attachment security can also help the therapist grasp how partners experience their relationship. The Relationship Questionnaire (Bartholomew & Horowitz, 1991) offers partners four sentences to endorse, using a continuous 7-point scale. These four sentences are designed to reflect partners' prototypical way of thinking about dependency and attachment. It is important, if this measure is used, that clinicians not think of it as signifying personality traits, but as an indicator of current ways of engaging specific significant others and dealing with dependency needs (Johnson & Whiffen, 1999). As previously discussed, there is evidence that the majority of trauma survivors who have been traumatized in the context of a close relationship have a fearful-avoidant perspective (Shaver & Clark, 1994). The therapist should expect such a client to be highly ambivalent about depending on another.

Depression co-occurs with marital distress, insecure attachment, and PTSD, and so, in general, it makes sense to assess depression when working with couples who are struggling with PTSD. Depression is increasingly seen from an interpersonal, contextual viewpoint (Joiner & Coyne, 1999) and related to the nature of an individual's attachment to others (Anderson, Beach, & Kaslow, 1999; Whiffen & Johnson, 1998). Shame about one's body has been found to be particularly predictive of depression and to mediate the relationship between depression and abusive experiences (Andrews, 1995). Depression is also increasingly being treated with drugs alone, in spite of evidence that, on the whole, therapy is more effective (Duncan, Miller, & Sparks, 2000).

Most often, the couple therapist will be able to consult with an individual therapist concerning the survivor's trauma symptoms. Measures such as the Symptom Checklist 90—Revised (Derogatis, 1977) can provide information on functional impairment and symptom severity. It has been difficult, however, to create a general test to assess PTSD symptoms that applies to different traumatic stressors and populations. The PTSD Symptom Scale Self-Report (Foa, Riggs, Dancu, & Rothbaum, 1993) is most appropriately applied only to victims of sexual assault, for example. An analysis of all the measures used to assess PTSD is beyond the scope of this book, but can be found elsewhere (Newman, Kaloupek, & Keane, 1996; Wilson & Keane, 1997). Other self-report PTSD measures include the PTSD checklist (Weathers, Litz, Herman, Huska, & Keane, 1993), used mostly with combat veterans, and the Impact of Events Scale—Revised (Weiss & Marmar, 1997). This 22-item revised scale adds items on hyperarousal to the original items on intrusive symptoms and avoidance that constituted the widely used first version of the scale. Granted, such measures are relatively quick and superficial and depend on the survivor's being willing, first, to connect with and describe his or her symptoms and then being willing to disclose them to the therapist at the beginning of therapy. Nevertheless, such measures give the therapist useful hints as to the echoes of trauma a particular client is dealing with and can provide material that can then be expanded in a therapy session.

The most widely used PTSD interview is the Clinician Administered PTSD Scale (Blake et al., 1990). This is a 30-item interview designed to evaluate the frequency and intensity of individual PTSD symptoms and related symptoms such as depression. Although the couple therapist may not be sufficiently familiar with this instrument to administer it him- or herself, it is useful to know whether a client's individual therapist has conducted the interview and to ask the client's permission for that therapist to share the results. The presence of serious personality disorder is often considered a contraindication for relatively brief treatments such as couple and family therapies (Gurman, 2001). Most often when such disorders are present, survivors do not seek couple therapy.

The most frequent exception to this is, however, the number of clients who do request couple therapy who have at some time been formally diagnosed as borderline. It has been suggested by trauma experts (Chu, 1998; van der Kolk, 1996) that this diagnosis is frequently associated with severe childhood trauma and that it reflects survivors' posttraumatic stress and the terror induced by depending on another after such abuse. In many cases, the diagnosis itself has exacerbated the survivor's sense of shame and helplessness and her relationship difficulties (interestingly, I have never seen a male diagnosed this way). Women who are angry, labile, and anxiety provoking are seen as "difficult" by health professionals and tend to be labeled as such (Chu, 1998). Herman (1992) has suggested that the term *chronic posttraumatic syndrome* should be used in place of borderline. I have found, all else being equal, that if these survivors difficulties are normalized in terms of fearful-avoidant attachment, they are often able to make good progress in couple therapy. The greatest stumbling block to such progress is often the survivors' sense of being "crazy and bad" and therefore deserving of abuse and unentitled to love and caring. Another problem that may occur, albeit very rarely, is that a client may exhibit not simply the numbing and avoidance common in trauma survivors, but the extreme fragmentation of a dissociative disorder (van der Kolk, van der Hart, & Marmar, 1996). Such a client has little chance of being able to engage in couple therapy as described here. If there is any question of such a disorder, the symptoms of which are amnesia, depersonalization or detachment from self, identity confusion, and derealization in which the present or the environment seems unreal or unfamiliar, the therapist may employ the Dissociative Experiences Scale (Bernstein & Putnam, 1986), to gain a clearer picture of this phenomenon, and refer the client for individual treatment.

If an attachment injury or a relational trauma is the issue, we have also used the Interpersonal Relationship Resolution Scale (Hargrave & Sells, 1997). This 44-item scale measures the extent to which a partner who has been hurt by another continues to feel pain as a result of the offense and has come to forgive this person for the offense. We have found it useful to employ this instrument at the beginning of therapy to help make attachment injuries explicit, and after termination to give both the couple and the therapist a sense of closure and completion.

Formal tests are mentioned here as constituting only one element of assessment, an element that can help the therapist quickly tune in to the key issues a couple or individual is facing, communicate and connect with other professionals, and find a way into difficult issues with a particular couple. Assessment can also be completed without any such instruments. Couple and family therapists have become particularly aware of contextual and cultural issues, and the aforementioned measures do not generally take such issues into account, although the field of trauma treatment has been attempting to address this concern (Manson, 1997). These issues discourage systems-oriented therapists from relying too much on such formal tests and encourage therapists to frame the echoes of trauma in an individual's cultural context. I have learned that it is best to frame a trauma in the language of the couple. Thus, a Native American (or First Nations) couple might speak of a "wounded spirit," whereas an English couple might speak of "our little problem" or a couple who read science fiction and history might speak of "facing the dragon."

In the assessment of trauma, safety and the therapeutic relationship are particularly important, so speaking to the individual therapists who have treated one of the partners over time is often more useful than asking the couple to complete a number of tests. It is particularly important to link with other therapists, because couple therapy is most often only one piece in the healing puzzle, albeit for some couples a crucial piece. Such consultation gives the couple therapist a sense of previous progress, dilemmas, and victories. The best assessment procedure for the couple therapist is most often the sensitive interviewing of partners, both jointly and individually. The couple therapist's perspective is also specifically focused on how the echoes of trauma affect each partner's sense of relatedness and responses to the other, and how relationship distress perpetuates the impact of trauma. This is a complex story, of which measures of relationship distress or individual symptoms can tell only a small part.

THE PROCESS OF EARLY SESSIONS

The majority of partners will disclose traumatic incidents in the first few sessions, even though they may not always directly link the impact of trauma to their present responses to their spouse. Once the therapist has seen the couple long enough to establish the nature of the dance in which the couple are caught, an individual session for each partner tends to strengthen the alliance with the therapist. Such sessions also allow for a preliminary exploration of any traumatic experience and its present impact on the relationship. Much of what occurs in these sessions resembles the early sessions of other collaborative approaches to couple therapy in general (Freedman & Combs, 1996; Wile, 1981), as outlined in the literature on EFT (Johnson, 1996; Johnson & Greenberg, 1992).This process includes explicating each partner's complaints and frustrations, listening to the story of the relationship and how the couple decided on couple therapy, piecing together from the partners' story the patterns in their dance, clarifying the strengths in the relationship and in each partner, observing and tracking the patterns in interactions, and taking a brief relationship history. The therapist is also creating an alliance and formulating the goals of therapy with the couple.

The key focus for the couple therapist in the first few sessions with traumatized couples is to get a sense of how coping with trauma and its aftermath has restricted the survivor's ability to connect with significant others and placed particular demands on the couples' relationship. Another piece of the picture is how the other partner's responses have contributed to the general distress in the relationship and may also have made it more difficult for the survivor to cope with his or her trauma and its aftereffects. It is important to ascertain not just how the survivor has learned to cope with traumatic stress, but whether such stress has also created secondary trauma in the other partner, above and beyond the distress of being in an unhappy relationship. Secondary trauma arises from having to deal with the traumatized partner's symptoms, such as unpredictable fits of rage or extreme hyperarousal and sensitivity to any kind of uncertainty or change. These symptoms are particularly distressing if, as seems to be most often the case, this other partner does not have any understanding of PTSD (Waysman, Mikulincer, Solomon, & Weisenberg, 1993) and so has no framework for understanding his or her spouse's behavior.

In early conjoint and individual sessions, the therapist and the couple create a coherent story of the relationship, the traumatic experience, and the connections between the two. Such a story may be summarized in the following manner: A male spouse "rescues" his wife from an intensely abusive family and the ghosts of her past. The couple then have a brief "honeymoon" in which they experience closeness and caring. However, when the wife suffers an accident and experiences chronic levels of pain, and then tries to commit suicide in response to a crisis in her family of origin, her husband is overwhelmed and feels personally rejected. So he withdraws from her. This withdrawal elicits desperate, angry responses from his wife and endangers the relationship. The tension in the relationship also exacerbates the wife's posttraumatic stress symptoms and results in their referral to couple therapy.

At this point in therapy, most couple therapists, no matter what their orientation, would be concerned with creating a coherent narrative that compassionately integrates the trauma in one person's history into the couples' experience of the relationship and the evolution of marital distress. Such a narrative may offer the couple a perspective, a platform from which to view the process of relationship repair, and a way of seeing their experience that does not blame or indict any individual, but makes sense of the experience. The organization of the experience is inherently calming and helps partners begin to regulate their emotional distress. The therapist has to move from listening intently and piecing together information, to organizing and validating the couple's present reality in a way that offers both partners hope and comfort. It is particularly important to formulate the dragon, that is, the terror and helplessness elicited by the trauma, and the negative cycle of interactions, often fueled by this terror and helplessness, as the problem. Survivors most often blame themselves for what has happened to them and can become caught in particularly vicious sequences of self-derogation concerning the potential failure of their marriage. The coherent narrative developed with the therapist offers an alternative perspective, but will be effective only insofar as the partners emotionally connect with it and make it their own.

INDIVIDUAL SESSIONS

The goals of individual sessions at the beginning of couple therapy can be summarized as follows:

1. To join with the individual client and hear his or her concerns in a context in which the other spouse does not have to be considered and is not a witness to the process.
2. To explore the individual's experience of relatedness in a way that does not automatically require this individual to confide in the other partner. This may help the therapist to refine the goals of therapy. For example, a partner may explicitly ask for assistance in telling her partner that she regularly dissociates during sexual activity.
3. To allow the therapist to probe difficult issues more sensitively, for example, drug and alcohol abuse, violence in the relationship, self-harm and sexual issues. The presence of violence between partners, a general contraindication for couple therapy, should always be determined (see Bograd & Mederos, 1999, for an excellent guide).
4. To allow clients to explore issues they cannot or are afraid to explore with a spouse present—for example, their present level of commitment to the relationship.
5. To allow clients to ask the therapist questions and voice reservations about therapy that they may not access or cannot admit to in front of a partner. For example, a partner needed to express how injured and blamed she had felt in couple therapy in the past, and her fears that this process would be repeated. She stated it this way: "You will see my husband as the shining prince trying to deal with the wicked witch. Therapists always do."
6. To allow for the concentrated exploration of particularly crucial issues without the concern or distraction of the other spouse's presence. For example, a survivor may not be willing to reveal the details of self-injury in the presence of the other, and the therapist needs to concentrate on these behaviors and the meaning of such responses in order to assess safety issues and formulate treatment goals. A spouse may also be unwilling to discuss issues of secondary traumatization in the presence of the other

because he or she believes it will further destabilize the survivor partner.

7. To set the stage for the couple sessions. As a result of the more concentrated intrapersonal focus in these sessions, the therapist can summarize the survivor's fears about trusting attachment figures or construct images of the trauma and its meaning, which can facilitate the process in future sessions. The non-traumatized spouse can also be given support and a way of understanding his or her partner's behaviors that will be useful in future sessions.

8. To allow the therapist to elicit further details about previous and ongoing therapy and attempts at coping with the effects of trauma and relationship distress. This helps the therapist relate the task of helping the couple build a more supportive relationship to the growth of the survivor and his or her taming of the dragon.

A further task of the couple therapist, as well as constructing with the couple a sense of where they have come from, where they are stuck, and where they are going with the therapist, is to educate the couple about trauma. For the survivor, this often involves clarifying and normalizing how this person's encounters with the dragon explicitly play out in the relationship and create specific needs and longings, as well as conflicts and fears. For the other partner, it may involve a more concrete discussion of the nature of trauma and its impact on its victims. The most powerful way to offer such information is in response to cues and events as they unfold in ongoing sessions. This is when new understandings are most meaningful. However, it can also help in early sessions to offer partners a basic definition of trauma and how it affects close relationships, perhaps in the form of easy-to-grasp images. These images can normalize both partners' responses and help them to empathize with each other. Thus, a therapist might talk about how blaming oneself for a trauma, especially for sexual abuse, is a universal and originally self-protective response, which then leads one to hide from others in shame and feel unentitled to being cared for. A therapist should also elucidate the fight, freeze, and flee responses to trauma cues and assist the couple to articulate how these responses specifically help create the cycles in their relationship. These dialogues help the couple to conceptualize the enemy they face and begin to clarify how the dragon steps between them.

It is worth noting that even for survivors who have been involved in extensive individual therapy and feel that they have integrated their traumatic experiences on a personal level, as couple therapy proceeds, these experiences are again assessed and redefined. Chu (1998) suggests, "Traumatic events are often experienced with an intense sense of *aloneness*. It is only with the support and sense of connection with another person that the events and all the attendant feelings can be tolerated, retained and integrated into memory as past experience, rather than remaining a dissociated psychological time bomb that is waiting to explode into consciousness" (p. 35). Once survivors begin to experience their attachment figures, their partners, as standing beside them, new and temporarily distressing memories, meanings, and feelings may arise. However, this is precisely because there is now hope of a secure base from which to deal with such memories, meanings, and feelings.

Given that assessment is not separate from treatment and that the clinical picture will be more complicated in some couples than in others, in general, by the end of the fourth session (two of the four being individual sessions) the therapist should be able to offer the partners a clinical picture or review that summarizes what she or he has learned about this couple and their interactions, the trauma and how it impacts their relationship, and each partner's strengths. The therapist can then relate all these learnings to the couple's specific treatment goals. Often at this point, a clear perspective on the problem and a sense of direction has already generated a sense of renewed hope and a de-escalation of negative interactions.

After such a summary, treatment goals can be reviewed by the couple, as well as their expectations of the therapy process. Thus, at this point in therapy, both partners and the therapist are defined as collaborators and traveling companions on the path toward more secure attachment and a relationship that can help the survivor heal.

Chapter 5

Interventions

The majority of traumatized couples who seek therapy are already aware that they are attempting to build a relationship in the shadow of the dragon. Most often, the trauma survivor is, or has been, involved in some form of individual psychotherapy to address trauma symptoms. As suggested previously, the couple therapist may then consult with the survivor's individual therapist, often the person who has referred the couple for therapy. The couple therapist focuses on how the trauma, which has already been named and delineated, plays a part in the negative interactions that characterize the couple's troubled relationship and creates blocks to positive and potentially healing interactions. The trauma and the ways of coping with it become part of the systemic formulation of the couple's relationship problems.

In many respects, early sessions with traumatized partners resemble first sessions with any distressed couple. As discussed in the previous chapter, the therapist's tasks are to create an alliance with both partners and to clarify their goals for therapy as well as their perception of the problems that face them. The therapist then gives an overview of the therapy process and reaches an agreement with the couple about what therapy will involve and how it will proceed.

There may be cases, however, when the survivor has confronted a trauma in individual therapy but the survivor's partner does not understand the impact or the specific nature of this trauma. Most often, the survivor has not felt safe enough to confide and openly communicate these issues. The sharing of such information may also then become part of the beginning stages of couple therapy and may continue all through the therapy process.

BEGINNING THERAPY: SPECIAL ISSUES

Even if the trauma and its effects on individual partners and the couple relationship are already well recognized and specified, there are certain elements of beginning sessions with traumatized couples that differ from the first few sessions with other distressed couples.

First, establishing an alliance with the survivor may take a little longer and require a little more care than is usual with nontraumatized clients. The therapist has to be particularly sensitive to the quality of the alliance with this client and must monitor it continuously, recognizing that survivors tend to feel particularly vulnerable and wary of placing their trust in any therapist. The alliance must also be more *explicitly collaborative*. To promote a sense of safety, it is important for the survivor to have a sense of control over the pace and direction of therapy. The therapist must strive to maintain a systematic, empathic attunement to both clients and to make the leap of imagination required to inhabit each client's world at key moments. Most recent models of couple therapy stress the need for such a respectful, collaborative alliance as a prerequisite for successful therapy (Freedman & Combs, 1996; Johnson, 1996). The quality of this alliance is even more crucial in treating traumatized couples, because issues of trust and safety are so significant.

Second, the symptoms of relationship distress are often more extreme than in other distressed couples, whose responses do not have the weight of traumatic experience behind them. Sexual problems, for example, may involve the complete cessation of lovemaking for a period of years. The survivor's extreme ambivalence about risking close connection with another may also result in confusing and apparently bizarre responses. For instance, a survivor may absolutely refuse all presents and tokens on birthdays and holidays, but becomes numb or explosive when his or her spouse stops offering them.

Third, the trauma may be relatively contained, perhaps as a result of having been dealt with in individual therapy, or it may not. The therapist must therefore be prepared to help clients deal with traumatic experiences that emerge in therapy sessions and must know how to help clients manage and contain their distress. The therapist occasionally has to engage in the basic tasks of trauma therapy with clients, focusing on, naming, and normalizing newly accessed or revived traumatic experiences that emerge as a result of the powerful interactions between the partners. Indeed, *the dragon is particularly likely to be reawakened at times when clients begin to take new risks with their partners.* For some systemically oriented couple therapists, these suggestions may appear to be too focused on the survivor as an individual. However, clarifying the partners' emotions and how they are expressed and communicated to the other spouse allows the therapist to link individual and system, the structure of inner experience and interpersonal response patterns. For example, when the partner of a survivor is supported to truly grasp, perhaps for the first time, the reality of the survivor's struggle to trust in the face of terror, the partner is often moved and wishes to reach out to his or her spouse. The survivor, at this stage in therapy, however, very often distrusts this response and cannot open up to the spouse's caring. This kind of event allows the therapist to draw a picture of how the survivor's fear and distrust compel him or her to push the partner away, even when that partner is trying to be supportive. This, again, leaves the survivor alone and discourages and exasperates the partner, making it harder for that partner to be responsive next time.

Fourth, as mentioned in the previous chapter, the therapist also has to be particularly aware of the survivors' ways of dealing with their symptoms that are destructive to them. At the very least, such coping mechanisms can undermine progress in therapy; at worst, they can make therapy dangerous for clients. The abuse of alcohol or drugs, behaviors such as self-mutilation, and suicidal ideation are common among survivors. These issues have to be explored. The therapist must ask the question, How does the survivor contain the impact of the trauma as it arises in his or her daily life? If the survivor cannot turn to the spouse for support, what does he or she do? The potential for violence is also high in survivors' relationships. Violence may take various forms, and the therapist should sensitively, but routinely, inquire about the possibilities. For example, survivors may routinely hurt themselves to exit numbing states or may become abusive to their children. A disproportionate number of survivors, especially survivors of childhood sexual abuse (CSA), are women. However, the number of male survivors coming into therapy seems to be increasing. There is, perhaps, a greater tendency for male survivors to direct their anger toward others and for female survivors to direct their anger against themselves.

Fifth, the therapist has to expect particular difficulties in general affect regulation and in the process of emotional engagement between partners. The therapist must note and explore sudden breaks and shifts in emotional reactions and in interactions between partners. The therapist may note, for example, the exact moment when a survivor exits from anger and sadness and becomes flooded with shame or withdraws into detachment and disassociation. The negative interactional cycle in traumatized partners is usually more complex than in nontraumatized distressed partners. For example, the couple presented in Chapter 7 do not follow a relatively simple pattern of pursue-withdraw. Both explode at times and both also withdraw at times. In general, because attachment needs are higher and, at the same time, emotional engagement is experienced as more dangerous, the steps toward more emotional engagement are smaller and there are more frequent blocks and impasses in the process of change. Couple therapy for traumatized partners may therefore have to be offered over a longer time period and integrated with the process of change in individual therapy sessions. Emotionally focused couple therapy (EFT), for example, is usually completed in 12 to 15 sessions even for seriously distressed couples. A number of couples who were dealing with complex PTSD resulting from childhood abuse or combat traumas (these cases are presented in Chapters 6, 7, and 9) were seen in a marital and family clinic in a general hospital for approximately 30 sessions. Other couples, whose problems were more circumscribed (the cases presented in Chapters 8 and 10), were seen for approximately 15 sessions.

ASSUMPTIONS UNDERLYING INTERVENTIONS

In general terms, couples who face dragons have taught me the following:

- Interventions must focus on and actively deal with the emotional experience that has control precedence (Tronick, 1989) in attachment situations and in responses to trauma, which tends then to override other cues. An attempt to bypass or marginalize emotion in dealing with attachment relationships and trauma is like leaving the fish out of fish soup. Therapists must help clients create a *working distance* from emotion (Gendlin, 1981), which is best described as being in touch with, but not overwhelmed by, an emotion. This is particularly important for trauma survivors who tend to either underregulate or overregulate emotion.

- Emotional responses cue relevant cognitive schemas and models of self and other, and these models are most effectively changed through corrective emotional experiences, rather than, for example, didactic reasoning, insight, or abstract, cognitive reframes or narratives.
- Attachment offers a powerful context for understanding and healing trauma and insecurity; thus, attachment needs and fears must be addressed.
- The therapist is an active consultant to the couple's relationship who is able to foster specific responses that interrupt both the interactional cycles that maintain trauma symptoms and the trauma symptoms that constrict interactions.
- The therapist will need to set specific interactional tasks, such as confiding fears about the unlovable nature of self, that step-by-step shape accessibility and responsiveness and so strengthen the bond between partners.

Within the context of existing models of therapy, the interventions described here will reflect collaborative models of intervention and a postmodern approach to change. Insight into the past may be part of the process in any therapeutic session, in any model. It is particularly useful to use past events and experiences to validate the self-protective stances partners take in the present relationship. For example, a therapist may comment, "Yes, of course, it is difficult for you to speak up here. From what you have told me, in your other family relationships there was very little safety and for you to speak up would have been very dangerous indeed. So it's natural now for you to shut down and retreat when things get difficult." However, what is most pertinent in couple therapy with traumatized partners is engagement with more adaptive forms of emotional experience in expanded and newly constructed interactions, in the present, with the partner. For example, survivors move from irritability or numbness, which alienates their partners, to clearly expressing specific emotions, especially fears and the needs associated with them, in a way that helps partners become more supportive. The validating stance of the therapist that is described here will be familiar to many therapists, particularly to humanistic experiential and narrative therapists. However, systems-oriented therapists who concentrate on restructuring interactions may be less familiar with a strong focus on such validation and on restructuring emotional experience. In fact, a focus on creating a secure base in therapy and on emotions and emotional communication is easily accommodated within the theoretical framework of systems theory (Johnson, 1998).

As mentioned briefly in Chapter 2, therapy can be conceptualized in three stages: (1) stabilizing the relationship and creating a secure base, both in therapy sessions and gradually in the relationship, (2) restructuring the bond between partners, and (3) integrating changes into the relationship and both partners' sense of self.

STAGE 1. STABILIZATION

There are two tasks for the couple therapist in the first stage of therapy: first, to create a safe context, and second, to clarify the couple's interactional patterns, their dance, and how the effects of trauma and a lack of security with the spouse shape these patterns. The overall goal is to deescalate the cycles of distress and to stabilize the couple's relationship. The therapist can then begin to shape this relationship as a potential safe haven and secure base, where both partners can find respite from traumatic stress. The following paragraphs discuss the two tasks in this first stage of therapy and the specific interventions used in each.

Stage 1, Task 1. Creating a Safe Context

This task involves the following:

• Actively creating a secure base in the sessions where partners can confront the ways in which trauma has defined their relationship and, often, their sense of self. The therapist must then strive to be not only affirming, but transparent. He or she has to be willing to be seen and not to hide behind the mask of professionalism. A client once stated, "Sometimes I hate you, because you see me. But then, I can stay here, 'cause sometimes you let me see you too."

• Reflecting and validating experiences that are poorly defined and marginalized. The therapist may validate the helplessness and secondary traumatization of the partners of survivors, for example. Such partners see only the shadows of the dragon, but they feel the fire of his breath nonetheless. The therapist must be able to do this while keeping a meta-perspective and honoring how such validation may be experienced by the other traumatized spouse. An attachment perspective fosters a nonpathologizing, normalizing approach to both the symptoms of deprivation and insecurity in the relationship and the symptoms of trauma that arise from living in a dangerous world without a safe haven. The reflection of marginalized experience and the affirming stance of the therapist encourages partners to engage in the therapy process.

• Collaborating with the couple in the formulation of safety rules and personal limits when such rules are necessary to increase the safety in the relationship. As specific trauma cues become clear, the couple can decide how to minimize their impact in the present relationship. For example, a husband is usually quite willing to modify his behavior once he understands that particular behaviors, such as his kissing his wife on the mouth, are direct trauma cues that make it difficult for her to respond to him. His wife is also much more willing to be physically close once he reassures her that he will respect such sensitivities.

• Beginning to educate partners about the interpersonal aftereffects of trauma as and when they appear in their relationship. Such education begins to cast survivors and their partners as dragon fighters. This offers a respite from the shame that most survivors slip into, even after successful individual therapy, when they begin to confide more specific problems associated with the trauma to the one whose disapproval they fear most, their spouse.

It is impossible to overemphasize how important alliance building is at this stage of therapy. Such an alliance is an ongoing construction, rather than a "once made, then stable and predictable" relationship. The therapist has to consciously tune in to and stay in tune with the couple in each session. However, so much is going on that missed steps and out-of-tune moments are inevitable. In fact, it is unlikely that therapy can be completed and the partners' vulnerabilities addressed without occasional breaches in the alliance. Thus, the therapist must actively monitor the alliance and be willing to give priority to mending it when necessary. In particular, the therapist must actively encourage clients to express their reservations and questions about the therapy process and must be able to respond in a nonreactive manner when challenged or tested. At one point a client stated, "I needed to push you a little to see if you really were as safe as you look."

The therapist should particularly expect to be challenged when addressing sensitive material for the first time—for example, when validating the nontraumatized partner's difficulties in dealing with the negative cycles in the relationship or with specific behaviors of the survivor (the survivor may hear this as blame). As suggested previously, it is important to explicitly respect the survivor's pace and to set a framework that invites feedback, during the sessions, about the process of therapy. The therapist may say to a client, "If at any time I ask you to put things into words or express things to your partner that seem too hard or scary at that particular moment, please tell me and we will find another way."

The therapist also needs to be realistic about the power of therapy and to talk openly to the couple about their expectations. Therapy cannot slay the dragon, but it can help to tame the beast and confine it to a small cage in one corner of the house, leaving other places for the couple to be close.

Specific Interventions for Creating a Safe Context

The main interventions that predictably create safety within a session are *empathic reflection, validation, empathic inference, and collaborative problem solving about safety issues.* It is perhaps not even accurate to imply that the first two responses are techniques as such, in that they represent a therapist's genuine stance toward clients. They are techniques in that they are deliberate, learned, and reflect a particular attitude toward clients and the change process. They are not techniques inasmuch as they reflect the self of the therapist who enters into a genuine encounter with each client. In this sense, the basic tool of the trade is the self of the therapist. Who you are and your willingness to engage with clients is the basic "intervention," especially with clients who struggle with existential vulnerabilities on a daily basis. At the beginning of therapy it is important to be discovery oriented. This involves being with each partner in his or her experience of the relationship, rather than immediately trying to modify symptoms and change patterns.

REFLECTION

Reflection has many functions, the most obvious of which are these:

- To create an atmosphere in which clients feel listened to and affirmed, and so free to explore and experiment.
- To check the therapist's understanding of client's experiences and allow the client to correct the therapist, if necessary, and so create a sense of partnership.

- To allow the therapist to sensitively direct the session toward the most salient topics and issues, bringing some elements to the fore and connecting them and letting others become background.
- To pace the session and allow the therapist to repeatedly zero in on key experiences and perceptions. Reflection slows things down and invites clients to "taste" and further process emotionally loaded information.
- To order experience so that it is less overwhelming and more easily endowed with meaning.

Particularly at this point in therapy, the therapist reflects and, in the process, better organizes emotional responses, perceptions of self and other, salient emotional issues, and the nature of traumatic incursions into the relationship.

Example

"You are talking about lots of topics here, about how you help with the house, about how you don't agree with your wife's view of your contribution to your life together, but the phrase you used a few minutes ago, the phrase 'Somehow I can never win here, it's hopeless. I can't take your pain from the past and make it better,' seems to be the main gist of what you want to say here. Is that right?"

VALIDATION

The accepting stance of the therapist is expressed in active affirmations of both clients' struggles, hurts, and fears. This intervention also has many functions:

- Validation increases the client's sense of acceptance and security in the session.
- It offers a positive perspective on each client's struggles and difficulties and so fosters hope.
- It normalizes both the problems arising from the trauma and the couples' relationship distress and so encourages engagement in the therapy process.
- It modifies the negative sense of failure and shame survivors often carry with them by modeling a compassionate, affirming way of seeing and responding to the self of each client.

The therapist actively takes the stance that both clients have many strengths and are in the process of growing. He or she particularly marks and elaborates positive ways in which each partner has coped with difficulties in the past and is coping in the present.

Example

"I understand that you feel you should be able to ask your spouse for what you need. But my sense is that your ability to shut down and tune out your needs saved your life in your family. So it's natural that you do that here. Especially when it's so new for you to feel safe enough to listen to your longings."

EMPATHIC INFERENCE

At times, even in early sessions, the therapist goes with clients to the edge of their articulated experience and tentatively unfolds and expands this experience. Although the client is the final arbiter of the nature and meaning of his or her experience, therapists are able to offer such expansions because of their knowledge of relationship patterns and the effects of trauma and because of their empathic attunement to the client's experience. The therapist begins to link and integrate into a coherent image each partner's emotional responses and inferences, which often echo traumatic experiences, as well as their interactional responses. The therapist always encourages clients to correct, modify, and clarify any inferences that he or she offers. The best inferences are simple, concrete, and encapsulate the client's present relational stance.

Example

"So, can you help me? I think I hear you saying that you are not only ambivalent about trusting here, but one part of you rebels at the very idea and says, 'Don't be a fool, you promised yourself, never again.' Is that it?"

COLLABORATIVE PROBLEM SOLVING ABOUT SAFETY ISSUES

The therapist actively probes for recurring events and issues that pose safety hazards or may undermine the process of therapy. Questions that focus on how partners deal with compelling negative emotions or recurring distressing events may uncover self-destructive behaviors, as revealed in, "I just get out on the freeway, hit the gas real hard, and tell myself I don't care anymore." Such questions may also uncover behaviors that alienate or terrify the spouse, as in threats such as, "If you go out tonight, I'll take all the pills in the cabinet upstairs." The therapist may help this client to articulate the core emotional message in such a statement, saying, "You are trying to get him to understand how desperate you are, and threats sometimes seem like the only way to do that." The therapist then focuses the conversation on the effects of such coping mechanisms on the couple's relationship and on the therapy process, encouraging the couple to agree on some alternative ways of calming and soothing themselves in specific stressful situations. The problem posed by such behaviors is viewed as one that is shared by both partners and the therapist, who all wish to prevent incidents that could derail the change process.

The therapist may also include basic education about the effects of trauma, particularly for the benefit of the nontraumatized spouse. For example, normalizing the survivor's need to withdraw at specific times, and linking this response to trauma cues arising in the relationship, can be a revelation for the other partner. Such partners, even if they have had some exposure to general information about trauma, are usually unaware of how specific trauma cues play out in their relationship, and most often take the survivor's coping responses as a personal rebuttal or slight.

Issues of safety within the session are also addressed. For example, the therapist may reassure a client that if a session becomes too distressing, the client has the right and means to take control and change the direction of the process. Therapist and partners may then discuss exactly how that would happen and how the therapist would respond. The process of therapy should be made as predictable as possible. At any time, the therapist should be prepared to meta-communicate with partners about the purpose and objective of particular interventions so that the process of therapy is *conducted with* the couple rather than *done to* the couple.

Example

"It sounds as though these threats to leave the relationship may offer you a way out of scary situations, an escape route, but then they poison the relationship between you and keep everything tense for days. Can we look at those situations and see whether we can find another way to make them less overwhelming, so you don't need to threaten each other this way?"

The interventions discussed so far are used *throughout therapy*. They are stressed here because they are particularly crucial in the first stage of therapy. In using any kind of intervention, how it is delivered is at least as crucial as the intervention itself. *A soft tone of voice and slow pace of delivery, for example, can make a reflection not only a structuring and ordering intervention, but also a soothing intervention that helps partners regulate their anxiety and other difficult emotions.*

Other interventions for expanding or reconstructing inner experiences that may be used in early sessions, but are used more extensively in later sessions, are elaborated in the following sections of this chapter. These include *evocative inquiry*, whereby the therapist asks *how* and *what* questions that focus on the leading edge of each partner's experience. These inquiries may concentrate on different elements of this experience—for example, on the cue or stimulus that sparks an emotional response, on exactly how this response is felt in the body, on associated desires and meanings, or on the action tendency primed by the emotion (as fear primes flight). The therapist may thus focus on the elements of an emotional experience and then summarize a partner's experience in the following way: "So as your wife smiled at your friend that way, the way she once used to smile at you, you felt your chest get tight, as if you couldn't breathe. Then you remembered that feeling of betrayal—the one you talked about as being always in the background around women. And then all you remember is feeling light and numb and finding yourself in the park hours later. Is that right?"

The therapist can also use a *heightening* intervention (although this intervention is used more often in later sessions), in which emotions are highlighted by repetition or imagery and their significance elaborated. The therapist may say, "When you see that look on her face, you say to yourself, 'Here comes the storm—there is nothing I can do.' And you just want to run, to find some way to escape. On one level you know she is desperate but you feel so battered that you just want to run away till she calms down. Is that right? (*Client nods assent.*) Can you tell her about that, please?" *Empathic inference or interpretation* (already mentioned, but used more extensively in the later stages of therapy) allows the therapist to offer partners new elements to expand their experience.

In terms of reconstructing interactions, the therapist expands and restructures interactions by *tracking, reflecting, and reframing interactions* and *setting interactional tasks* that restructure the way the couple interact around attachment issues. In early sessions, the therapist will most often simply reflect the patterns of interaction presented by the couple in their descriptions of past events, and in their interactions in the present, and ask them to make these explicit. In general, because fear and helplessness narrow awareness and constrict experience and interaction, the therapist attempts to expand and restructure how experience and interaction are constructed.

Stage 1, Task 2. Clarifying Interactional Patterns and the Emotional Responses That Shape These Patterns

This task has three elements:

• To track and identify the negative interactional cycles that maintain the distress in the couple's relationship. These cycles of attack and alienation reflect and cue absorbing states of attachment insecurity in both partners. They also make collaborative problem solving, effective affect regulation, and mutual soothing impossible.

• To begin to specify how the emotional responses of both partners in their attachment dance reflect the impact of trauma and attachment insecurity. For example, an extreme need for sexual contact may arise when a male survivor is constantly ambushed by reminders of the shame and helplessness he experienced as an isolated and abused child. As a result of his demands, his wife becomes overwhelmed and moves away from him, confirming his worst fears. The survivor may already have clarified in his or her individual therapy the legacy of trauma and the particular attachment sensitivities that arise in the relationship. However, sharing such sensitivities with a partner and experiencing in the here and now the specific role they play in sabotaging closeness, is another step. The partner also needs support to share the experience of attempting to create a relationship in the shadow of the dragon. The therapist slows the interactional dance and points out that, at key moments, it is the specific attachment insecurities and echoes of traumatic stress that dictate the steps.

• To help the couple form an overview of their interactional patterns and emotional responses in a way that empowers them and helps each partner to view the other as an ally in a common fight, rather than as an enemy or the main architect of the problems in the relationship.

The best outcome of the first stage of therapy is a de-escalation of personal and relationship distress. Negative relationship cycles slow down and become less automatic. The couple begin to have a meta-perspective on these cycles and the part trauma plays in them. Each partner can see the whole picture of the drama that is the relationship and how his or her moves in this drama affect the other spouse. They begin to move together in the battle against their common enemies—the cycle and the trauma embedded in it. Moreover, they begin to see each other as a resource in this battle and the relationship as a potential safe haven.

What does this haven look like? From an information-processing, cognitive standpoint, the couple use fewer blaming attributions and show more ability to look at the relationship as a whole and to acknowledge the part each plays in the creation of distress. From an emotional standpoint, the partners are less volatile, more positive and hopeful, and are more able to explore their own emotions, particularly the "softer" emotions such as fear, shame, and sadness. In terms of interactions, the couple are more open, more engaged, and more able and willing to confide.

Specific Interventions for Clarifying the Partners' Interactional Cycles and Underlying Emotions

TRACKING AND SUMMARIZING INTERACTIONS

The therapist tracks and reflects key interactional events and patterns and summarizes these patterns into a coherent drama. He or she listens to the story of the couple's relationship across time and the more detailed descriptions of specific, significant episodes, and watches how the couple interact in the session. The therapist can then track the process of positive and negative interactions and reflect the patterns that emerge. *How the couple communicates and moves in relation to each other is the focus, not so much what they talk about.* The sequence of interactions is reflected back to the couple, and recurring patterns are delineated and named *in collaboration with them.* The formulation of the cycle is, at best, in the partners' own words and phrases. It is a joint construction, with the partners giving the raw data and the therapist helping to link elements and organize the construction. The formulation thus captures the clients' experiences and so is easily owned and used. The therapist also helps the couple piece together a coherent narrative of how these patterns evolved and any key incidents that solidified or elaborated them. He or she then helps insecure, distressed partners to do what secure individuals do naturally—that is, reflect on and create coherent narratives about their relationship and events in that relationship, and move to meta-processing and meta-communicative levels. Partners can then see and discuss patterns and put responses in an interactional context.

It is also important to listen for exceptions to negative patterns and highlight times when the couple were able to deal with problems in ways that fostered safe emotional engagement between them. It is as if the therapist were holding up a mirror and saying, "Is this the dance? When does it move into steps that hurt and paralyze you, and when does it pick you up and bring you together?" The therapist replays and summarizes interactional sequences to make them visible and clear.

The couple are invited to stand back and look at the cycles that define their relationship negatively and make both of them vulnerable to the dragon and his fire. The therapist identifies such cycles as maintaining the distress and insecurity in the couple's relationship and victimizing both partners, defeating their attempts at contact and caring. A typical cycle may be as follows: criticize and protest followed by defend and distance, leading to increased criticism that ends either with an explosion by the distancer or long periods of mutual withdrawal. Such cycles are characterized as having "run away with" the couple's relationship. When the couple enact their dominant patterns in the session, the therapist highlights and summarizes the process and encourages the couple to outline the negative effects of such cycles. If exceptions to the pattern occur in the session, the therapist also comments on these and asks the couple to explore what made such responses possible.

Example: Tracking and Unfolding Specific Moments in the Interaction

"What just happened here? You turned your head, and he began to talk about your 'sensitivities.' Is this one of those times when you just want to 'shut him out,' as you put it?"

Example: Sequencing Key Interactional Events and Summarizing into a Coherent Drama

"Is this what always happens now when he does risk and reach? You are so unsure, you reach for your yardstick and comment on where he has failed, and he gives up and moves away again. Is that it? So you push for closeness, but when he offers it, it's so hard to trust, you can't quite take him up on the offer. And I guess [*to the other partner*] you get confused and discouraged then and just stay away?"

REFLECTING AND EXPANDING UNDERLYING EMOTIONS

Once the cycle has been described in a manner that resonates with the couple, the therapist begins to *reflect and unfold, with tentative evocative inquiries and inferences, the underlying emotional responses* and *frame them in the context of attachment insecurities and the echoes of trauma.* The therapist does this by specifying and giving form and color to marginalized and avoided emotional responses. He or she sensitively infers their attachment significance and begins to bring these emotions into the dialogue with the partner. Once the nature of the underlying emotional responses is tangible and clear, the therapist may *heighten* them to bring them to center stage.

As they occur in the session, the therapist focuses on emotional responses and places them in the context of unmet attachment needs and attachment fears. For example, when Carol's face flashes with rage at her partner's rational remarks, she closes her lips and goes silent. The therapist tracks and unfolds the elements in this vivid moment, noting Carol's angry expression, her closing of the lips and turning away. The therapist then helps Carol to articulate and explore her rage, rather than become overwhelmed by it or avoid and deny it. As Carol then actively connects with her rage, the therapist stands beside her and supports her processing and organizing of this experience. The therapist then continues to ask evocative questions that encourage a deeper engagement with this experience. New elements then emerge. In this case what emerges is a "sense of outrage" at her partner's seeming indifference to her pain. This client then begins to experience a deep sense of aloneness that fuels and maintains her rage. This aloneness has a conceptual element ("No one will ever be there for me") and an immediate emotional element ("I feel so small, and no one will ever come and hold me"). It is linked to the original experience of trauma and abandonment and the sense of disconnection in Carol's present relationship. Carol then begins to recognize and engage with the pain of her isolation and the terror associated with it. She begins to recognize that in her rage, she pushes Jack, her partner, away when she needs him most.

Clients like Carol are supported to specify any links between her present sensitivities and her past traumatic experiences. They then begin to be able to listen to the information inherent in their emotional experiences. Emotions tell us about what is important to us and what our needs are. As such clients organize their inner emotional experiences differently, as they listen to a different music, they naturally place their feet differently in the relationship dance. The therapist encourages Carol to tell Jack directly about her aloneness and her sense of his inaccessibility, evoking an engaged emotional interaction in the here and now of the session. (Sometimes a client can talk to the therapist about his or her emotions but finds it very hard to turn and tell a spouse, even though the spouse has just heard the information in the dialogue with the therapist. The therapist is safer to engage with.) Carol's expressed pain pulls her partner toward her and evokes his compassion, encouraging him to risk a greater level of emotional engagement. The therapist can then integrate this client's sense of desperate aloneness, linked to and exacerbated by specific trauma cues, and her implied need for reassuring contact, into the story of the interactional cycle.

The nontraumatized partner also has an opportunity to explore and share how the shadow of the dragon has constrained the relationship for him or her and, in many cases, has evoked secondary traumatization. For example, the therapist focuses on specific nonverbal emotional responses of Carol's partner, Jack. He compulsively swallows and blinks at times when Carol criticizes him. As the therapist reflects these nonverbal responses and asks evocative questions, he then begins to explore his experience of his wife's anger (see the following examples of interventions). Partners like Jack often know the facts of the past trauma in a cool, cognitive way, but do not understand the heat of the survivor's experience and the way it is evoked by present interactions. They also need to have their own emotions recognized. For example, they may need to express their resentment at being the "fall guy" and bearing the brunt of their traumatized partner's anger or hostility. One such spouse remarked, "Before I can hear her, I want her to get how she lashes out at me. I've made lots of mistakes, but I don't think I deserve all that rage." Even if they feel empathic, they often have no sense of how to respond effectively to the onset of the cycle and their partner's intense affect. The therapist normalizes these partners' coping strategies, such as the tendency to minimize the trauma experienced by the other, and helps them to begin to understand the survivor's distress. The therapist also identifies this partner as a potential source of comfort, an ally, who can help turn the tide in the fight with the dragon. These partners most often respond with relief to the knowledge that they can play a positive and crucial role in their partners' healing and the healing of the relationship.

Examples: Expanding Experience with Evocative Inquiry

This intervention offers the therapist a key method for clarifying and deepening emotional realities. The therapist asks concrete process questions, that is, *what, how,* and *when* questions, focusing particularly on painful, deep feelings, such as sadness or fear, that are normally avoided or lost in more explicit reactive numbing or irritation. The therapist goes to the edge of the client's experience as presently formulated (as much as is possible in beginning sessions) and asks the client to take just one more step (Johnson, 1996; Johnson & Denton, forthcoming).

"What is happening to you right now, when, as you describe it, he looks 'bored'?"

"You sound angry, but you have huddled down in your chair. How does that feel, to hold your arms close around you like that?"

"You used the word 'mysterious' to describe your partner. What happens to you when he seems 'mysterious'?"

Example: Expanding Experience by Heightening Marginalized or Barely Processed Responses by the Use of Images and Repetition

"So, can you help me, Jack? Your blinking comes with a sense of confusion, yes? It's as though all you can do is blink. Is this one of those times when you go all 'still' and 'frozen'? Carol is mad. You have 'blown it' and the storm is coming. Is that it?"

Example: Expanding Experience by Linking Trauma and Attachment Cues to Specific Interactions and Cycles

"Right there, Carol, when he reached with his hand, is that one of those moments when alarm bells go off and you get caught between longing—stepping forward—and the sense of danger, the same sense of danger you had when you were small, the danger in putting yourself in his hands?"

Example: Expanding Experience Further by Encouraging the Confiding of Newly Formulated Responses

"Can you tell him, 'I long to let you hold and comfort me but it feels so scary, so I step back and test you'?"

"So, can you tell her, Jack, in a simple way, 'I hear what you are saying and I want you to risk with me. I'd like to learn how to comfort you'?"

By the end of the first stage of therapy, the couple's negative interactional cycle becomes explicit and more manageable and the couple less disoriented and overwhelmed. They are also more hopeful and engaged with each other. The couple have the beginnings of a secure base from which to tackle Stage 2 of therapy.

STAGE 2. RESTRUCTURING THE BOND BETWEEN PARTNERS

In Stage 2 the therapist collaborates with the partners in three tasks. First is the restructuring of the partners' emotional experiences in the relationship, and second is the use of new emotional experiences to revise the partners' associated sense of self. Third, the therapist sets interactional tasks to bring these new experiences and identities into the relationship in a way that creates new and more positive interactions by the partners. Negative responses are gradually replaced by new responses that foster accessibility and responsiveness, the building blocks of a secure bond. All the interventions used in Stage 1 (described above) are also used in this stage when appropriate. However, there is a greater focus on heightening and empathic inference to shape new responses and the setting of interactional tasks to shape new interactional cycles.

Task 1. Expanding and Restructuring Emotional Experience

The restructuring of emotional experience involves claiming and congruently expressing a partner's avoided or as yet unformulated experience, and integrating it into that partner's sense of self and the dialogues that define the relationship with the other partner. Partners are now safe enough in the session to touch and own the ways they protect themselves, and to explore the fundamental fears and insecurities that constrain them in their relationship. As they do, they clarify their attachment needs and engage with their partners in a new way.

For example, in previous sessions a withdrawn spouse may have been encouraged to look beyond the "numbness" he experiences when his traumatized partner becomes enraged to and articulate the "uneasiness" that sparks his disengagement at crucial moments in the dance with his partner. At this point in therapy, the therapist will encourage him to explore this uneasiness further. As he recognizes the tightness in his chest, and the voice in his head that tells him he is a wimp and a failure, he finds himself weeping. He is able to integrate these thoughts and feelings, and he expresses his experience as "total intimidation." This emotional experience, when it is owned, encourages him, indeed literally moves him (the word "emotion" comes from the Latin *emovere*, "to move"), to take a stand with his wife. The therapist helps him formulate his stance and to engage his wife from this stance. He tells his wife that he cannot tolerate her recent rages and that he longs for the times when he felt comfort and closeness with her. As he expresses this ever more forcefully, his habitual way of engaging his wife begins to shift. He becomes more accessible and more assertive. His sense of self also changes, because he sees himself, as the narrative therapist would say, enacting a preferred identity. He experiences himself as more competent and more in control, and indeed he is. When his wife then bids for attention in a testing way, he can stay engaged. This interaction expands the possibilities in the couple's dance.

At this central stage of therapy, when partners are more fully engaged with their emotions and often discovering elements of those emotions for the first time, there may be times when the therapist helps particular partners, especially survivors, move between emotional exploration and the containment of emotion. In general, being supported to put experience into words, order it into a sequence, and have it heard and accepted by another, in and of itself allows a client to feel a sense of control. If the experience becomes overwhelming, however, and the client loses his or her way, the therapist can provide a coherent focus and help this client contain the experience.

For example, if the client is dealing with a flashback and is becoming sidetracked and disoriented by flashes of shame, the therapist may help the client to stay focused on his or her fear. If the client becomes immersed in intense distress, the therapist can actively help the client to regulate his or her affect by reassuring, reflecting the experience and placing it in the context of present safety. The therapist then acts as a voice-over, slowing, summarizing, and containing the experience and connecting the client to concrete experience in the alternate, present reality. The therapist may reassure the client, "You are here with us, and this is what is happening. You are safe now. Can you feel your back against the chair?" It is also important to support clients' attempts to soothe themselves, such as by taking deep breaths and moving physically into a comforting, protected position. A specific example of this kind of emotional containment can be found in the literature (Johnson & Williams Keeler, 1998).

In general, however, clients in the second stage of therapy can permit more intense emotional experience to emerge in response to the therapist's evocative inquiries, heightening, and inferences. They can also explore this experience more actively, accessing in a new way, for example, a sense of shame and articulating the fear of exposure and the need for acceptance that this implies. Emotions are the signposts to our most significant desires and needs, and at this stage in therapy, emotional experience evolves and is regulated and organized differently. Fear may, for example, evolve into longing or grief. New emotional experience orients people to their attachment needs and allows them to send clear emotional signals to the spouse in a way that motivates the partner to respond.

Example: Expanding Experience with Evocative Inquiry and Reflection

"What happens to you as he reaches for you? Can you look at him? What do you see in his face? You said he seemed as if he was a long way away."

Example: Heightening Core Emotions and Attachment Responses So Clients May Grasp Their Significance

Heightening is best done in simple, concrete language and images.

"Part of you says, 'It's so foreign and strange to hear that I am precious to someone—that he values me—that he doesn't think bad things happened to me because I was somehow at fault.' It's hard to grasp that. [*Client nods.*] Your feelings of shame tell you it can't be true. You don't quite know how to take it in, how to react. So you stand very still, frozen. Is that okay—am I getting it? [*Client nods.*] Can you tell him . . . ?"

Task 2. Expanding Self with Other

The restructuring of one partner's emotional experience in relation to the other involves collaborating with partners to integrate newly formulated emotions and new responses into a new sense of self. Contacting marginalized or disowned emotions and integrating them into ongoing experience expands each partner's sense of self. As a partner listens to different emotional music, he or she then steps differently in the relationship dance and acts in a way that fits with his or her new experience. Thus, the husband described earlier sees himself being more assertive and feels more confident and empowered when his wife responds to his new sense of self. When he experiences himself as competent and more capable, emotional engagement with his wife is not only possible, it is exhilarating.

This is particularly significant part of the process of therapy for survivors. These partners' sense of self, especially in the context of close relationships, may be less well integrated, less coherently organized. A client once remarked, "Different parts of me want different things, and I sort of swing between them." The self is also more negatively defined in these partners than in nontraumatized partners. Survivors may access intense shame at this point in therapy. Such emotions tie into denigrating self-schemas that frame the self as unlovable and deserving of rejection and even abuse. Once articulated and owned, emotions of this kind can then be countered by the empathy and acceptance of the therapist and, more important, the empathy of the other partner. The other partner's responses, which become more caring and compassionate, act as an antidote to the survivor's negative sense of self and provide a new corrective experience of affirmation and comfort. As Berger and Luckmann (1979) point out in their seminal book on the social construction of reality, significant others are the principal agents in the maintenance of that crucial element of subjective reality called identity.

The therapist focuses on and heightens statements that point to a more positive emerging sense of self. He or she also clearly marks and normalizes conflicting responses and places them in the context of traumatic stress so that they become more coherent. Denigrating self-schemas are framed as the natural consequences of past hurts and traumas in which others have been malicious or indifferent and so have acted as if this person were inconsequential or deserving of abuse. The therapist choreographs interactions that evoke alternative, reassuring responses from the other partner as to the lovable nature of the survivor's self.

Example: Expanding the Self by Heightening Positive Elements of the Self

"You have no picture in your mind, no image of what it looks like, how it feels to be really safe in someone's arms—but you find your courage, follow your longing, and you keep fighting, testing, and trying."

Example: Expanding the Self by Reflecting and Ordering Emerging Elements of the Self to Promote Integration

"The wounded part of you just wants to close up and keep everyone out, but the fighter part of you still wants to risk—is that it?"

Example: Expanding the Self by Reframing and Offering Alternatives to Negative Self-Images That Arise

"You see her as toxic, that little girl who was you? You don't see how strong she was, how she fought to survive even though she was all alone in the dark."

Example: Expanding the Self by Fostering Confirming Interactions with the Other Partner

"Can you help her with those feelings? Can you tell her how you respond when she says that she isn't worth fighting for?"
"Can you hear him when he tells you that he needs and wants you and wants to comfort you?"

Task 3. Restructuring Interactions toward Accessibility and Responsiveness

At this point in therapy, the therapist also explicitly and more actively restructures interactions to facilitate more secure bonding. As a result of clarifying their emotional experiences in the manner described above, partners can now directly own the interpersonal stances they take in the relationship and their consequences. Thus, a survivor can now tell his or her partner, "Yes, I do shut you out. I do it with my silences. And then I test you really hard to see whether I can risk letting you in, and, of course, you fail. Then I don't have to risk it." Couples naturally use images of connection and disconnection (e.g., shut out) to capture the quality of their contribution to the dance. At this stage the individual's focus is more on the way he or she habitually engages the other and how this defines the dance, rather than on the other partner and who is to blame for the couple's distress.

As a partner reshapes his or her emotional experience, moving perhaps from anger at the partner and the self into a new sense of grief and helplessness, the therapist reflects the new emotional experience in a simple, brief summary and invites this partner to share this experience with the other. *New engagement in inner emotional experience then translates into new signals sent to the other and a new kind of emotional engagement with this partner.* The therapist supports this kind of sharing by empathic reflection and validation of the risk involved in confiding. He or she also helps the other spouse to listen. The therapist effectively engages partners in experiments in new kinds of interactions, interactions that have potential to build trust and security in the relationship.

If a partner cannot risk connecting emotionally with the other spouse, this difficulty is explored as it occurs. The therapist may take a short detour and suggest that such a partner tell the other how hard it is to risk, and focus on how the other can help him or her begin to share. The therapist may even validate that this person cannot share at the present moment and then ask how that block to sharing is experienced. Similarly, if a spouse has difficulty responding, this is explored on a process level. In terms of timing, it is important to prepare a previously withdrawn and unresponsive spouse and help him or her to re-engage before encouraging the other spouse to become vulnerable and take risks.

When new kinds of interactions do occur, especially if a partner shares personal vulnerabilities and the other responds with caring, the therapist will reflect and heighten this response. The therapist frames such responses in terms of their attachment significance, pointing out, for example, that a spouse is leaning forward and looking concerned, as if he wishes to comfort and protect his wife. The therapist then enlarges the screen and calls attention to the effects of these new kinds of interactions and how they may strengthen the relationship and empower the couple in their fight against the incursions of a trauma.

Events in which the survivor is able to reach out for help and support to deal with trauma symptoms or attachment insecurities are particularly noted. Events of this kind have been found to predict recovery from relationship distress for couples in therapy (Johnson & Greenberg, 1988) and are particularly important for traumatized couples. These events generate trust and offer an antidote to the violation of connection that is the essence of many traumas, especially traumas that give rise to complex PTSD. They also create an alive, compelling experience of the couple relationship as a safe haven. As discussed in previous chapters, once the relationship is defined as such, there is a viable escape from helplessness and a constructive way to regulate affect and trauma symptoms.

> *Example: Increasing Responsiveness by Heightening More Responsive Interactions*

> "He is offering to comfort you. He is inviting you to come and let him take care of you. Do you see him?"

> *Example: Increasing Responsiveness by Inviting the Partners to Risk More Engagement*

> "Can you turn your chair, look at him, and tell him what you need right now?"

At the end of the second stage of therapy, the couple are actively creating positive bonding cycles in their relationship and are much more intrapersonally and interpersonally in control of the fight when the dragon emerges from the dark. They fight together against the hopelessness and helplessness that is the essence of trauma, and every time they fight the dragon together, the bond between them grows. Moments of extreme vulnerability and stress seem to have the ability to define and redefine realities. Sartre noted that strong emotion involves a transformation of the world. When the dragon comes, there is no room for ambiguity. You are either with me or against me. If suddenly you are with me and I see that, then this changes everything. It changes how I experience myself and my vulnerability, how I experience you, and the nature of the bond between us.

Impasses in Therapy

The most common point at which the process of change tends to become bogged down is toward the end of Stage 2, particularly when the survivor begins to take significant new risks with his or her now emotionally accessible partner. Often, if the therapist affirms the difficulty of learning to trust after trauma and remains hopeful and engaged in the face of a temporary reoccurrence of distress or distrust, the couple will continue to move forward. Specific attachment injuries may, however, arise and have to be addressed (see Chapter 10).

The therapist may also set up an individual session with each partner to explore an impasse and soothe the fears associated with a new level of emotional engagement. The therapist can also reflect the impasse and invite the couple to reclaim their relationship from the cycle and the dragon. Heightening and enacting an impasse can also be useful. For example, a survivor actively articulating her stuck position in the relationship may feel the constraining effect of this position more acutely. So, sadly stating to her partner, "I can never let you in. If I do . . . ", can begin to challenge this position. The partner too can often respond in explicitly reassuring ways that allow the survivor to take small new steps toward trust.

If emotional reactivity is very high and interferes with any kind of intervention, the therapist can offer images and tell archetypal stories that capture the dilemma of the survivor and the partner. The couple are then able to look at themselves and their interactions from a distance and explore such a story, slowly moving closer to engaging with the dilemmas in their relationship (Millikin & Johnson, 2000).

STAGE 3. INTEGRATION

Integration occurs on three levels: self-definition, relationship definition, and each partner's resilience to traumatic stress. The first task is for the therapist to help integrate newly processed emotional experiences and new self-schemas into both partners' sense of self. Thus, a survivor may remark, "I have been wounded and trusting is hard, but I can risk and I am worth loving." The partner may state, "I can step outside the spin we get into now, and I think I can be there for her, and that makes me feel strong again." One such partner stated, "Well, if she is facing dragons, maybe sometimes I can even be her hero and help her fight them off. You need heroes around dragons."

The second task is for the therapist to integrate new kinds of interactions into the couples' definition of the relationship by reflecting and heightening new interactions and their significance for the nature of the bond between partners. A survivor may say, "There will be hard times, but I know I can reach out for him now, and he'll comfort me. I'm not all by myself in the dark." The therapist may heighten such a remark by bringing up instances of how this husband comforted his wife and talking about exactly how she reached for him and what now made this possible. Third, the therapist ensures that new ways of coping with the ghosts and scars of trauma are explicitly integrated into models of self and into the relational system. Thus, a survivor says to her husband, "I know I can lean on you when those old memories come for me. I don't have to be ready to fight for my life every time. Knowing I can lean on you makes me stronger, so that, often, I don't even need to come to you."

The change in the survivor's relationship now endows him or her with a new resilience that protects this person from relapse when new stressful events arise and potentiates the gains made in other modalities, such as individual therapy. Studies of anxiety disorders, such as PTSD, tell us that the responses of close family members are the most powerful predictors of the maintenance of treatment benefits (Craske & Zoellner, 1995). Every time the survivor is able to turn to her spouse for soothing and comfort, the positive cycle of trust is affirmed and the hold of the debilitating effects of isolation, terror, and attachment insecurity are lessened

Integration on the aforementioned three levels is achieved by *reflecting, affirming and heightening new positive interactions and bonding events* and *constructing empowering narratives of the change process*. More secure emotional engagement is now possible, and the therapist also *supports the couple in problem solving difficult issues* that have divided them in the past.

Constructing an Empowering Story of the Change Process

The therapist helps the couple construct a simple, cohesive narrative of the process they have been through in therapy, detailing where they started and where they are now. This story includes an affirming account of how they changed their relationship and now deal with the echoes of trauma differently. The therapist reflects present, positive cycles and frames them within an attachment context. It is particularly helpful to support partners in formulating a version of the story of change that stresses their efficacy and competence in healing their relationship and dealing with the dragon. The couple are encouraged to discuss their expectations for the future and the continued growth of their relationship. Narrative therapists who focus on exceptions to client's problems and systems therapists who heighten enactments that constitute alternatives to problematic patterns will be familiar with such interventions.

Fostering Pragmatic Problem Solving of Divisive Issues

The couple are now able to use their problem-solving skills with minimal support and direction from the therapist. Once the fear arising from the traumatic experience and relationship insecurity can be comfortably regulated in a manner that contributes positively to the growth of the relationship, the couple can effectively use all the problem-solving skills in their repertoire. Clinical experience and research on EFT interventions have shown that people do not generally need to be taught such skills. Once they have increased the safety in their relationship and no one's toes are dangling over a cliff, they are able to see the other's point of view, to be clear about their needs, and to formulate effective solutions. Those who experience a felt security with attachment figures are generally able to consider alternative perspectives and to better engage in collaborative problem solving (Kobak & Cole, 1991). At this point, the couple can engage each other in new ways and solve the pragmatic problems that every couple has to deal with, such as parenting and finances.

The therapist encourages partners to be realistic and to plan for the time when the dragon again rears his head, as he surely will. The partners problem solve around anticipated future difficulties and ongoing differences between them, such as the survivor's need to restrict sexual activities or how to handle recurring triggers such as anniversary dates.

Heightening Bonding Responses and Events That Define the Relationship as a Secure Attachment

The therapist observes the couple's interaction and takes any opportunity offered to foster bonding interactions and heighten their significance. The therapist validates positive new ways of coping with insecurity and trauma symptoms that arise in the session and in the couple's account of their life at home. He or she encourages partners to continue to confide their attachment needs and fears to each other and to elaborate on the responses the partner makes that each finds soothing and reassuring. The therapist invites the couple to describe explicitly how the relationship now meets their needs for a safe haven and a secure base.

Finally, the therapist and the couple discuss the termination of therapy and any anxieties of the couple about terminating. The couple are encouraged to turn to each other for support, rather than to the therapist.

Example: Heightening Positive Interactions and New Ways to Cope with Trauma

"I want to stop a minute and go over what just happened here. You started to feel that 'wooziness' that comes up when you know you are open to hurt. [*Client nods.*] But then you turned and told him about that, and he got up and held you for a few minutes. Isn't that one of the times when, in the past, you might have gone upstairs and taken all those pills?"

Example: Heightening New Definitions of Self

"So, when you courageously ask for help at those times, and he knows he can help, both of you feel more in control and both end up feeling precious and valued by the other."

Example: Heightening and Choreographing Repeated Positive Bonding Interactions and Heightening the Meaning of Such Interactions

"Can you tell her what it meant to you when she stood up for you with the doctor? Can you tell her how much it helped you?"

Example: Constructing Empowering Stories of the Therapy Process

"The two of you have come so far. I think back to the beginning, when it was so hard for you to put your weapons down and let each other in. But now you can turn to him and put yourself in his hands and let him hold you up. And you can support her and share with her your own fears and difficulties. What do you see as the key changes here, and how do you think you made them together?"

Example: Pragmatic Problem Solving

"Can you hear him when he says that he worries that your sex life together will stall and will not keep improving? I think you were trying to let him know some of the ways he can help you feel safe and positive with your sexuality, weren't you? Can you help him to understand more about that?"

By the end of therapy, the couple have created a safe haven to rest and heal and a secure base from which to learn and grow. When couples come for therapy, not only are they facing the threatened loss of their attachment relationship and the very real danger of fighting the dragon alone, but they constantly have to deal with the fact that any close contact with the partner may call the dragon forth. At the end of successful therapy the situation has changed. The appearance of the dragon is now an opportunity to experience and affirm the power of connection between them. Facing dangers together builds strong bonds.

The following four chapters present four examples of couple interventions for trauma survivors and their partners. The cases were chosen to illustrate different kinds of trauma and couples entering therapy at different stages of dealing with these traumas. The background of each case is given, and key events in the change process are presented and discussed.

Part II

Clinical Realities: Couple Therapy with Traumatized Couples

Chapter 6

Couple Therapy to Create a Secure Base for the Treatment of Trauma

"If only there were less of me."

T he majority of couples dealing with trauma in their relationship are referred to or request couple therapy after the survivor has spent some time in individual therapy, at least enough time to delineate the trauma and contain some of its effects. There seem to be two most frequent referral points. That is, referral most often occurs when the survivor's individual therapy reaches an impasse and the need for a more supportive couple relationship becomes clear, or when certain trauma symptoms have been dealt with but the powerful, debilitating effect of interpersonal symptoms that are maintained by relationship distress becomes apparent and must be addressed. However, a smaller number of couples also find their way to a couple therapist before the survivor partner has really started to address the trauma. For example, a social worker in a local hospital refers a client who has been hospitalized for repeated suicide attempts and whose spouse is seriously depressed. This client has managed to tell the social worker about her childhood abuse and her flashbacks, but has not been able to confide in her spouse. The client then enters couple therapy at the same time as beginning individual therapy for the first time. In cases of this type, the goal of couple therapy is to de-escalate relationship distress, create a secure base for the containment of symptoms arising from the trauma for both partners, and begin to make the couple's relationship part of the healing process. This process then also potentiates the survivor's individual therapy. In many cases the ultimate goal of couple therapy, the creation of a secure bond, will require that the survivor first address the trauma and its effects in individual therapy before engaging in couple therapy to address interpersonal trauma symptoms. This chapter explores couple therapy that occurs when the dragon is unrecognized and untamed. It discusses how to help partners come together in a way that helps the survivor turn and begin to face and fight the dragon.

THE CASE OF CHARLENE AND JIM: "IF ONLY THERE WERE LESS OF ME"

Charlene, 34, and Jim, 37, were referred to the couple and family therapy clinic in a major urban hospital by a psychiatrist who was presently treating Charlene for severe anorexia in an eating disorders clinic. Charlene was not making progress in the clinic, although she had received individual and group therapy for more than a year. The psychiatrist believed the reason for her lack of progress was that her marriage was in considerable distress. The couple scored 82 on the Dyadic Adjustment Scale. This is just above the cutoff score generally used in the clinic to differentiate severe from moderate distress (moderate distress = 80–90, milder distress = 90–100). On the RQ attachment measure, Jim showed a basically secure style, and Charlene showed a fearful-avoidant style. Jim had his own business and worked long hours. Charlene had not worked since a car accident 3 years earlier, which had resulted in spinal surgery and chronic pain. The couple had two little boys, 5 and 8 years old. Charlene described her days as dealing with the persistent pain in her legs, keeping a "perfect" house, attending the eating disorders clinic, and surfing the Web.

Both partners stated that although they were committed to their marriage, they no longer felt connected with each other. Jim spoke of a "lack of intimacy," and Charlene said, "We respect each other, but there is no Jim and Charlene. We are just roommates." Charlene saw these problems as beginning at the time of her car accident and the birth of their second child. Jim agreed that he had withdrawn more at that time as a way of dealing with Charlene's "irritability." When they described their present life together, their interactions seemed to fit into a chronic withdraw–withdraw pattern. Jim put in many hours at work and spent time with his children, and Charlene liked to spend time in her room with her computer. When I fostered interactions between them in an early session, however, their interactions took on a pursue–withdraw quality. Charlene became upset and tearful or angry at Jim's "distance"; Jim's face became very still and tight, and his sentences became shorter and shorter.

When I asked about how their relationship had evolved, and when it had been positive for them both, they responded that they had met 10 years ago, when Charlene was hospitalized for suicidal depression and anorexia. Jim had been visiting a relative in the next bed. They had quickly connected with each other and had, as Jim described, it a "fun, carefree relationship." Charlene had seen Jim as a "protector and a friend." Charlene also stated very calmly that intimacy, especially sexual intimacy, had always been difficult for her, perhaps because she had been sexually abused as a child. Charlene had not addressed this abuse in treatment for her eating disorder. The eating disorder, which had remitted after her first hospitalization, when she had met Jim, had reemerged about 2 years ago after the operation on her spine. She stated, "I have always had a body image problem. I can't undress in front of Jim, and sex is always difficult. I feel not wantable. So I started exercising and not eating." She attributed the beginning of her current anorexia to the fact that Jim's distance had reached a critical point for her, and her sense that she was undesirable. When asked directly by the therapist, Charlene also stated that when she and Jim made love, she would have vivid flashbacks of previous abuse and she had been able to mention this to Jim. As Charlene spoke of these problems, Jim began to weep. He said, "I knew bad stuff had happened, but we don't talk about it. I just thought she would get over it in time. I'd like to help her, but I don't know how." He also said that he had been keeping his distance since her treatment for anorexia began, because he had decided that it was best to give her space and not "trouble her"—and he did not know what else to do. Charlene said that she had experienced him as increasingly involved with the kids and less involved with her since her operation and her problem with chronic pain. He pointed out that she was irritable and did not seem to want him to come close to her.

This couple were easy for me to connect with. They obviously cared for each other. Charlene's swing between irritated pursuit and self-protective withdrawal seemed typical of an abuse survivor. Such clients often show fearful attachment styles, characterized by an intense need for comfort and connection and fearfulness about exposing the self and risking closeness. Charlene also spoke of the chronic pain in her legs and mentioned that she now tried to keep it to herself so as not to upset Jim. She also mentioned feelings of guilt because her chronic pain, and now her anorexia, prevented her from working and contributing to the family finances. Jim expressed sadness and loss and stated, "I watch every word I say. Since she had that accident, I feel that I lost my friend." Charlene also stated that she saw Jim's main priority as being a parent for their two boys. Jim repeated that he did not know how to help Charlene, and so he tended to "stay away," because showing his own confusion and distress would probably make her worse. Charlene then described herself as a "liability" and expressed the belief that she shouldn't be married at all. Jim replied that she was "precious" to him. When I asked Charlene to talk directly to Jim about her distress at the distance between them, she resisted and commented that they were now so far apart that talking directly to him about anything was difficult. She then said that she had survived in her life by becoming "invisible," and she knew that this was now a problem in her relationship with Jim. She felt that the only solution was to "get rid of as much of me as I can." Her husband wept.

The following salient points emerged in the next couple session and two individual sessions:

1. Charlene had grown up with a widowed, extremely physically sick mother, who had been unable to protect her from the violent sexual overtures of her step-brothers and cousins and the general hostility of the extended family, who disapproved of her mother and father's marriage. Charlene's much older cousin, who had taken over in the role of parent when her mother died, had been punitive, verbally abusive, and withholding of food.

2. Jim had also lost his father at an early age, which had connected him with Charlene. He, however, had a relatively stable and happy upbringing. He agreed that he had retreated into his work and parenting his boys as his connection with his wife had become more tenuous.

3. In her individual session, when questioned directly, Charlene stated that any sexual contact brought with it terrible flashbacks of abuse. She had shared "a little" of this with Jim over the years, but had "held lots of it in." A recurring flashback was of having plastic pushed over her face while being raped and being unable to breathe. She

downplayed her abuse and its effects, suggesting that lots of people had experienced this and were "doing okay." It was just that she was "toxic." What emerged in her story was that her leg pain, which her spouse saw as the main issue, was manageable for her. Her inability to eat and her withdrawal and aversion to touch, even with her children, seemed to directly reflect her traumatic past. Only if she initiated touch would she find it pleasurable. When asked directly, she spoke of intrusive flashbacks, numbing, and avoidance (not eating would create numbness and a sense of being at a distance from reality), alternating with flashes of rage and irritability. She would dress in the dark so as not to see herself, avoid touching her own body, and tell herself, "Everything will be fine if I am no trouble. So I will try to take up as little space as possible. It's best if I am invisible." She also spoke of herself as "damaged," "unwantable," as well as "toxic." However, she did not see herself as needing individual therapy and downplayed her trauma and the guilt of her abusers unless I asked specific questions. She did want to save her marriage. She described herself as confused about directions for change, stating, "I'm down so deep, I don't know which way is up. All I know is that I don't want to lose Jim." When I asked Charlene whether she had any questions, she asked if "this" ever went away. My answer was no, not entirely, but I had seen others face their demons and find a way to keep them in the margins of their lives rather than have to live their lives around them.

4. Jim described himself as keeping his distance so as to not lose his wife altogether. He knew the bare bones of Charlene's upbringing, but did not understand her present problems and responses as a reflection of this upbringing. He felt helpless and "stood still" so as not to "rock the boat any more." We discussed the pain and fear in Charlene's life and how he had, in some sense, lost her to it.

This couple's interactional pattern was clear, swinging between mutual withdrawal and Charlene's becoming angry and pursuing—up to the point of physical touch at least. As she described it, she would become numb and "go somewhere else" if touch became sexual. She did like being held if she felt "in control." This couple's strengths were that they clearly and honestly cared about each other and wanted their marriage to work. They spoke of the brief time before Charlene's first pregnancy as being blessed for both of them. They were also easy to connect with and engage in the therapy process. Considering the problems they were facing, they were not as distressed as they could have been. They expressed less blaming and criticism than many other distressed couples and could still comfort each other at times. This last element may have been the crucial one.

We set out the immediate goals of therapy: We had to find out how Charlene and Jim could stand together and bridge the distance that had come between them, and how to tackle Charlene's difficulty with nourishing herself in a way that would bring them together. We talked about the long-term goal of having a close, safe, stable relationship. To achieve this goal, we would need to discuss how Charlene's past violations at the hands of those she relied on sometimes flooded her with fear and shame and carried her off into another country where Jim could not reach her. I cast Charlene's trauma as a dragon that she had become accustomed to fighting all alone. Her willingness to risk connecting with Jim at all, after such a history, was described as spirited and heroic. Charlene would refuse this description, but smile profusely as she did so, and talk of the "dragon" while refusing to accept that she had experienced trauma. We described Jim as "defeated" by Charlene's distance, laboring under the dragon's shadow but not knowing how to grapple with it. I normalized Charlotte's need for reassurance and her fear of too much closeness, and Jim's guardedness and "standing still." We made a contract that we would meet once a week, and that if either partner began to feel increased distress, he or she could contact me. I also conferred with Charlene's therapist at the eating disorders clinic and shared the goals of couple therapy and my clinical impressions. I stressed that I saw Charlene's eating disorder as an attempt to deal with the echoes of trauma and that our plan was to help Jim become a resource in dealing with these echoes.

STAGE 1. STABILIZATION: PROCESS STEPS AND KEY EVENTS

We began the fifth session by outlining in more detail the "dances" that made up the couple's relationship. There was a positive dance of friendship and holding that sometimes came to "visit." There was a dance of mutual guardedness and distance, and a recurring dance of Charlene's becoming "enraged" and often "running away, before I hurt Jim or the kids" or showing her irritation. Jim sometimes then verbally "hit back" and "devastated" her. We focused particularly on times when Charlene could go to Jim for comfort and closeness, which was *when she needed it least*. If she was "drowning," she could not reach out. She said, "I'd upset him, add to his stress, and I am toxic—so I hide." This was more extreme than the usual lack of confidence in the other's availability and responsiveness displayed by distressed couples. First, Charlene did not feel entitled to caring and comfort; she felt compellingly unworthy. Second, she saw herself as dangerous, as contaminating her loved one. This sense of self as poisonous, rather than poisoned, seems to be specific to those who have been severely and intrusively violated by attachment figures. At some point, this blaming of the self may have been an adaptive alternative to acknowledging complete hopelessness and abandonment, or becoming angry at a dangerous or, as in Charlene's case, dying attachment figure. However, despite our myths of lone heroes battling demons, it seems to be that isolation and self-denigration elicit only more helplessness and feed the beast. Third, the risk involved for Charlene in reaching out when vulnerable was enormous. She wanted comfort, but some part of her also felt it was "disgusting." Jim also acknowledged that recently there had been times she did reach out and he was busy protecting himself and did not respond.

The partners' emotions and their steps in the dance, each creating the other, began to be made explicit. Both partners explored specific incidents, elaborated on past responses, and, most compellingly, engaged in interactions in the here and now that could be explored and clarified. The couple's drama then began to develop just as a picture forms in a tray of developing fluid. They were able to reconstruct the steps in their negative interactional pattern. Charlene formulated this pattern in the following terms:

- Jim shuts down rather than show her his frustration at her distance, her irritability, and her "refusal" to eat.
- She sees the frustration in his face anyway and remembers incidents such as the time when he called her a "basket case," confirming all her worst fears about herself.
- She then withdraws further, or angrily protests and then withdraws until she feels "invisible."

After hearing her description, Jim began to weep and was able to tell Charlene that he watched everything he said and stayed away so as not to hurt her. With my help he expanded this into sharing with her that he was "completely terrified" of losing her to her "sickness." I emphasized the irony here: He kept his distance precisely because she was so precious to him. Charlene saw his distance as proof of his rejection of her and her unworthiness and "hid" from him even more. Both partners began to "see" and "touch" how their attachment fears directed the dance and trapped them both in helpless isolation. I described Jim as frozen, paralyzed by his fear of losing his wife, and Charlene as in flight (occasionally lapsing into fight) from both the fear of closeness and the fear of loss and abandonment. The shadow of the dragon behind this drama became plain.

When I was able to focus Charlene on unfolding her experience of shame, she was able to identify the "voice" of hopelessness and self-denigration as echoing the messages of her cousin who had parented her after her mother died. Hearing this cousin's hostile voice in her head always preceded Charlene's "giving up" on Jim's loving her and moving into "invisibility." She also began to use the sessions to share with Jim more specifics about the nature of her traumatic experiences (she now accepted them as such) and her flashbacks and how they colored their interactions for her. This was difficult for Jim to hear, but also evoked deep empathy from him. He understood that Charlene had held back some of the specifics of her abuse from him over the years, but did not resent this. He intuitively knew what I sometimes explain to other spouses who do react negatively to the fact that the partner has kept secrets from them, namely, that, as Dostoevsky suggested, everyone has reminiscences that they tell only to their friends, but there are also things that a man (or a woman) is afraid to tell even to himself. These kinds of things are then usually not confided in others, even those closest to us. Jim began explicitly to validate Charlene's traumatic experience and her survivor status. Charlene found this very moving and wept as he affirmed her pain and voiced outrage on her behalf. With my help she began to see him as an ally against the dragon and the "voice of the enemy," that is, her cousin's voice and the part of her that accepted her cousin's denigration of her.

Jim and Charlene were now able to process and express a much larger range of emotions to each other in the session, and after a discussion of safety cues, we were able to come up with a daily comfort ritual (an intervention I have used with many survivors and their partners to increase safety in the relationship). In this case, it was a ritual of drinking hot cocoa together at night. At these times they could just "shut the dragon out and hold each other." They also found they could comfort each other in other ways, particularly if Jim made his approach slow and predictable and Charlene was able to still the "voice of the enemy" and allow herself to feel entitled to ask for the contact she wanted. They became more hopeful and were able to step out of their cycle of mutual withdrawal, at least some of the time. Jim also began to understand that "there is something I can do" and viewed himself as "standing with" his wife when old images, emotions, and voices caught up with her. The distress in the couple's relationship began to abate, and Charlene began to eat, at first only when Jim was not present and then with him. The couple's relationship and Charlene's symptoms began to stabilize. She also began to accept that she had been significantly hurt and might "deserve" individual therapy. The couple now actively referred to the dance they were caught in and the dragon in the shadows, rather than each suggesting that the other person was at fault for their dilemma. This can be seen as an example of a couple developing a "healing theory" (Figley, 1989). Jim also began to encourage his wife to seek individual therapy and to see herself as a victim rather than a "disease." As they were able to confide in each other and influence their relationship, they began to express more confidence and a sense of efficacy.

As a therapist, I had to work hard to stay focused on the pattern of interactions and the emotions embedded in them and to help the couple construct new dialogues. There was a temptation to become immersed in dealing with Charlene's dramatic images of trauma and self-blame and self-harm. I had to remind myself that I could not be an individual therapist for Charlene. My job was to help her create a safe haven with Jim, a platform where she could stand and face the dragon. We are naturally unwilling to risk such a confrontation if we experience ourselves as alone and vulnerable. We know that we are not designed to face dragons alone. Perhaps, as Bowlby (1973) suggested, "being alone, like conscience, doth make cowards of us all" (p. 147).

STAGE 2. RESTRUCTURING THE BOND BETWEEN PARTNERS

The couple now moved into the second stage of therapy, that of changing interactions to improve the bond between them. The most natural first step is to help withdrawn partners to become more engaged, or, in this case, because both partners tended to withdrawal, to help the one most able to be responsive and accessible to take that stance. With support, Jim began to move to a much more engaged stance. If we listened in at crucial moments in this process, what would we hear? What would these key events sound like?

First, Jim began to express his frustration and explicitly connect it to his longing for his wife. He said, "I feel alone too, you know. I come home and have to check—very carefully—about how much I can approach you. I need support too. When you recoil from me, it hurts. So then I do start to hold back." Charlene did not respond very well to this, suggesting to Jim that he "gave up" on her and that she was a "burden." I encouraged Jim to continue to speak from his heart and encouraged Charlene to hear him as struggling to be with her and fearing her rejection.

He said, "I want you to fight to be with me. I am not your cousin. I am not your abuser. I want you to let me in and tell me how to help you." Charlene wept at this and said she felt reassured, but then she turned her body away. She was able, with help, to tell him that she had flipped into anger after a few moments of relief. Her impulse was to say, angrily, "Keep your hands off me." We then began to talk about how much she needed control over others touching her. Later that week at a family funeral Jim was able to interject himself between her and one of her abusers. On one hand, she denied that she needed this ("I shouldn't mind. I should be over all this"). On the other hand, she expressed great relief at his support.

As Jim became more open and responsive, Charlene expressed less fear and began to become mired in shame, saying things like, "Don't waste your time on me. I'm raw—I'm not comfortable in my own skin—you need a lover, a wife." With a little support, Jim was able to stay engaged. He told her, "You don't get to decide whether I fight for you or not. I need you, and I will wait. And we will learn to be close in ways that you can feel safe. I'm not going anywhere." He also began to habitually identify the voice of Charlene's shame and self-denigration as the "voice of the enemy" and to respond to it by labeling it and offering his alternative affirming perspective. I supported him in this stance and helped him to stay focused and clear in his interactions with his wife.

All these responses constituted a new kind of engagement on Jim's part. His more present and responsive stance having been facilitated, the task was then to help Charlene to become more engaged so that she could at least elicit and use his support. It is at this point, as emotional engagement with the partner becomes a real possibility, that the echoes of trauma usually intensify as the survivor fully experiences the vulnerabilities associated with such a connection. For Charlene it became increasingly clear that she would need to confront the dragon herself before she could create a more secure attachment with Jim and be able, for example, to find sexual contact or other forms of close contact pleasurable. The goal was then to create the most secure base possible, and to stabilize the relationship and her symptoms as much as possible, so that she could engage in this process. The main themes that emerged here were the fear of closeness and difficulties with affect regulation in general, the risk involved in creating new trusting interactions, Charlene's struggle with self-disgust and shame, and how this struggle impacted the relationship. The last issue is a crucial one. How can one accept love if, to survive, one has had to give up on it and adopt a sense of self as unlovable? Consider the following session excerpt, in which the therapist is attempting to help Charlene risk taking some new steps:

THERAPIST (*to Jim*): You would like to comfort her. (*Jim nods emphatically.*) It feels sad not to be able to reach for her when you know she is hurting. [Therapist reflects his statement and infers his emotional state from his nonverbal responses.]

JIM: (*very softly, looking at Charlene, who is staring at the floor*) I'd really like to hold her, to help make it better.

THERAPIST: Can you tell her, Jim (*motioning with her hand toward Charlene*)? [Therapist structures interactional task.]

JIM: (*very softly*) Let me hold you, just let me be there. (*Stretches his arms out toward her; Charlene smiles, then looks doubtful and turns her body so her shoulder is toward him. She looks away.*)

THERAPIST: What is happening, Charlene? Jim is reaching for you, do you see him? (*Charlene nods.*) What is happening right now? [Evocative inquiry]

CHARLENE: I feel irritated. (*Glances at Jim and then turns to the therapist.*) See, he's crying now. I'm obviously toxic. He should stay away.

THERAPIST: When you see him reach for you, which is something you have spoken about with longing in previous sessions, right now you feel irritation and you feel afraid that you might hurt him? Is that right? [Reflection of emotions]

CHARLENE: Yeah. I can't handle nice things. My stomach twists. I have nowhere to put it. (*Jim weeps; she turns to the therapist.*) You see, I'm a disappointment no matter what!

THERAPIST: What happens to you when he reaches out and tells you that he wants to help? [Therapist stays in the moment and asks an evocative question.]

CHARLENE: (*long silence; she answers in a flat voice*) Don't know (*pause*). Well (*long pause*), I get this "ping" feeling . . . yes, . . . it's like . . . ping.

THERAPIST: Ping, hum, is that like alarm? (*Charlene nods.*) Do you believe him? [Empathic inference by the therapist.]

CHARLENE: No, so I'm mad. And yes, and it's scary. He might get close. He might want sex, and I'll disappoint him. I should be able to respond to him. I'm untreatable.

THERAPIST: So "ping" is anger. No one ever protected you, and Jim sometimes withdraws too. And "ping" is fear and hopelessness. People you have trusted have burned you. Closeness is just so scary, so the alarm goes off. [Therapist reflects, orders, draws simple, concrete inferences.]

CHARLENE: I should be over all this. I'm defective. I feel better giving to Jim. It's hard for me to, well, I don't like receiving.

THERAPIST: Aha. All this anger and fear. The "ping" comes and you can't take anything in, can't put food in your mouth or let Jim give to you, comfort you. It's all too scary. [Therapist reflects, draws inferences, and summarizes—focuses on Charlene's inability to accept comfort.]

CHARLENE: (*very quietly*) I want to crawl under the rug. I can't breathe. (*Grips the chair arm; her hands are shaking.*)

THERAPIST: (*speaking softly and calmly*) It's okay, Charlene. You're here, in my office. No one will hurt you here. This is so hard. You needed this alarm system, it probably saved your life. You so needed comfort, especially when your mother died and those who came close hurt you so badly, terrified you. All you could do was try to be invisible, hide, stay away, and get smaller. [Therapist moves to contain emotion, reassures, normalizes, and summarizes relationship stance.]

CHARLENE: Yes, not eat. The more I eat, the more I feel.

THERAPIST: Aha. And if Jim comforts you, and you let him come close and touch you, you will feel. And if you let him see you, it might feel like those other times . . . and so the alarm goes off. [Therapist reflects, summarizes.]

CHARLENE: (*Weeps and covers her face with her hands.*) My memory is tangible. I can still feel "his" hands on me. I can still hear "his" laughter, and I feel sick. The only way out is less of me.

THERAPIST: Was there ever a time when all this shame, and fear, and anger didn't step between you and Jim? When the dragon didn't step between? When there was another way out?

CHARLENE: In the very beginning maybe. I still trust Jim more than anyone. But if I feel upset, everyone is an enemy.

THERAPIST: So what would you like from him now, Charlene? [Therapist directs her back into the interaction, focuses on her needs.]

CHARLENE: I'd like him to be there and let me go through this. Be there, but not too close right now.

THERAPIST: You can't let him comfort you right now, but you want him to stand beside you while you look the dragon in the eye? (*Charlene agrees and nods her head.*) Please, tell him. (Therapist motions with her hand, sets interactional task—choreographs a specific kind of engagement.]

CHARLENE: (*Turns, makes eye contact with Jim, tears, and speaks very softly.*) Stand with me . . . can I ask you?

JIM: (*to the therapist, softly*) She is worth fighting for. (*Therapist motions with her hand toward Charlene. Jim turns to Charlene and whispers.*) You are worth fighting for.

CHARLENE: (*Smiles and turns to the therapist.*) He's my boomerang. He keeps coming back. He gives me courage.

JIM: It's easier, now that I understand what is going on. I do hold back . . . I'm sometimes . . . I don't know what to do, how she'll react. I get overwhelmed, kind of numb. But I'm here. I'm here for the long haul.

As this excerpt suggests, when Jim offers Charlene comfort and caring, the violation of human connection she has experienced prevents her from responding. Her fear, rage, and self-depreciating shame become an absorbing state, in which everything leads in and nothing leads out. Yet here, in the preceding sequence, she begins to name and order her shifting emotions and to ask for what she needs. As a therapist, I was aware of "holding all sides of the client's feelings, until she can hold them herself" (Grossman, Cook, Kepkep, & Koenen, 1999, p. 60). Charlene then went on to help Jim understand that accepting any kind of attention and relaxing into pleasure or a sense of comfort was "suicidal" when she was growing up. In light of this experience, it is a tribute to the human spirit that Charlene was able to connect with Jim and allow him to "rescue" her from her family of origin.

Jim was now consistently emotionally engaged and supportive in the sessions and in the relationship in general. The next step in the usual practice of emotionally focused couple therapy (EFT) would be to have Charlene risk being vulnerable and move significantly closer to Jim. As we talked about it, the three of us, we agreed that this was down the road a way, and that the task now was to identify the blocks to allowing herself to feel and communicate her needs in the relationship. In a nutshell, these blocks were the fear of closeness, which would bring up images of violation, and Charlene's shame and sense of unworthiness. She was also absorbed in the struggle with her trauma and what it meant for her and her life. Jim began to actively encourage Charlene to seek a trauma therapist who could help her to confront her flashbacks, her numbing and withdrawal, and the ways of seeing herself that arose from her past. He actively supported her when she had to have a medical exam, which was extremely distressing for her, and began to arrange for her to eat with him every day, even if it was just a snack. He was also able to share his frustration when his support (such as calling her beautiful) was also labeled by Charlene as threatening because it might lead to sexual overtures. With my help they agreed that for now, the rule was no sexual overtures or contact. This pragmatic problem solving around this sensitive issue then made holding and hugging more feasible for Charlene.

Charlene began to be able to share with Jim when she got stuck in negative thoughts and emotions, such as blaming herself for her abuse and even for her mother's death, and he would comfort her. Jim began to talk about how he felt less "lonely" and that it was a great relief for him for him to "finally understand what is going on" in his relationship with his wife. He stated that he had started to understand Charlene's "irritation" as part of her response to her past and not to take it so personally. The recurring themes during this time were first, Charlene's extreme ambivalence about closeness, how she would alternate between terror of abandonment and fear of being "exposed" and vulnerable, and how Jim would then become confused and frustrated; second, how interactions would impact each partner's sense of self; and third, the meaning of Charlene's traumatic experiences and how they created the "music" for this couple's dance. There were also moments when I had to stop and pay attention to the alliance between Charlene and me. At one point she told me, "I hate it when you zero in, and I hate it when you get him to say stuff directly to me." I did my best to honor her feelings, and we talked about how "foreign" such contact was to her and why there were times when I insisted on it.

Consider a final excerpt, which deals with Jim's explicitly joining the fight that Charlene was always waging, the fight about who she was and whether she was entitled to love and care.

CHARLENE: I have to keep a perfect house. If I forgot a chore when I was a kid, I would be locked out. My cousin said I was useless. So I clean and clean and clean.

JIM: You are more important to me than whether the house is spotless or not. (*Charlene shakes her head vehemently.*)

THERAPIST: That's hard for you to understand, Charlene? (*Charlene nods.*) It's kind of foreign. You never got that kind of message. Well, perhaps from your mother before she got sick?

CHARLENE: I'm not sure. I just hear such clear voices from back then— it's hard to let myself hope that what he says is true. (*Jim sighs, puts his head down, and rubs his forehead.*)

THERAPIST: That's hard for you to hear, Jim?

JIM: You bet it is. No matter how much I'd say I loved her, she would-n't accept it. (*Sighs, tears.*)

THERAPIST: What was that like for you, to offer your love but have Charlene unable to let it in? That must have been hard.

JIM: It really gets to you after a while. I'd feel helpless. Like nothing I did made a difference. I couldn't get through to her. So then, I guess, I'd withdraw. (*Turns to Charlene, speaks in a soft, quivering voice.*) I try to give you confidence, but it doesn't seem to count.

THERAPIST: How do you feel as you say this, Jim? You sound sad, or . . . ?

JIM: I pull back—I feel rejected, but, but its also, I feel like I'm being pulled down by her negativity, or I'd try to be sympathetic, and then she'd say she was just making mountains out of molehill, I couldn't comfort her either. (*Weeps profusely.*)

THERAPIST: Can you help me to understand, Jim? This brings up real grief, sadness for you, yes?

JIM: Yes, I can't reach her—and it's like I'm losing her. But I get scared too—I lost my dad, you know, like she lost her mom. I comforted my mom—I was only eight, but I was the man of the house. I comforted her.

THERAPIST: You dealt with your grief by comforting your mom. (*Jim nods.*) And it feels awful not to be able to comfort Charlene—to feel helpless and to be filled with grief yourself—fearing losing her and being drowned in all that loss?

JIM: Yes, yes, that's it. (*Raises his voice.*) And goddamn it, I want her to listen to me.

THERAPIST: Can you tell her, please, "I want you to listen to my voice, my voice telling you that you are loved and lovable." You want Charlene to begin to let in your voice and the other voices that cared for her—her mom, her aunt. You want her to not let herself be consumed by the voices of those who abused her. They told her lies about how who she was and what was happening to her. They told her it was her fault, that she was bad.

JIM: (*looking at Charlene*) Right, yes.

THERAPIST: Can you tell her, please? (*Motions with her hand toward Charlene.*)

JIM: (*Leans forward and speaks insistently.*) Listen to me—my voice counts—I am here.

CHARLENE: I want to, I want to hear you. I am starting to accept that what happened was really something—I want to struggle with it. If I listen, if I eat, if I hear you, I start to get mad—maybe that's bad . . .

JIM: I'd rather you get mad—I can deal with that.

CHARLENE: I am listening. I tell you things now, things I've never told anyone. I woke you up when I had that nightmare . . .

THERAPIST: You accepted the flowers he bought you, with a smile. (*Charlene nods and agrees.*) Can you let him know when his voice is helping you feel loved and is beginning to be heard over the things your abusers told you. (*Charlene nods and smiles.*) What does it feel like when you can hear his voice and let yourself, just for a moment, trust his message?

CHARLENE: (*beaming*) It's like rain in the desert. (*Therapist motions toward Jim.*) It feels like rain in the desert and it helps me fight—fight the dragon. It makes me think maybe I can even struggle with things like making love—if you love me.

This couple made considerable progress. By the end of therapy, they could eat together; Charlene was no longer consumed with shame if Jim saw her put food in her mouth, and her eating disorder was abating. She had begun to talk about her abuse in the eating disorders group and recognized that "I guess I have to touch the hurt to push it out of my life—or at least, to the side." Charlene started individual therapy to work specifically with her trauma and reported that she was making progress. Jim and Charlene would hold hands as they walked out of our last few sessions, and Jim stated that he saw her rage as part of the trauma and did not now become injured by it. He was more responsive to her, and she could tell him when she could be touched and when she had "no skin" and had to be alone. She could also break the one rule of survival in her family, which was "Keep your mouth shut," and tell him when she felt flooded with fear. She said, "I take little steps. The closer I get, the scarier it is, but . . . it's happening. I never really expected to be, well, attached. Thank God he's still here."

At the end of couple sessions, this couple's relationship was still, to a certain extent, defined by the echoes of Charlene's trauma. In terms of the process of change presented in this book, Charlene and Jim were not able to reach the same level of comfort and connection as other couples. Jim became re-engaged and more responsive, but Charlene still needed to protect herself from Jim and the terror that closeness evoked in her. For example, they were not having sexual contact, and Charlene was not ready to involve herself in the full emotional engagement and bonding events that are usually associated with the end of Stage 2 of therapy and recovery from relationship distress in EFT (Johnson & Greenberg, 1988). The sessions ceased by mutual agreement, so that Charlene could focus on her individual therapy, with the expectation that the couple would return at some time in the future to complete the work on their relationship. As usual in the final stage of therapy, I helped the couple to formulate a coherent, empowering narrative of their journey through therapy and how they would see the relationship continuing to improve in the future. This included heightening positive patterns of interaction and the impact these interactions had had on each partner's sense of self. As at other times, the couple were encouraged to enact in the session the new steps toward positive bonding they described in their narrative. So Jim talked about how he had told Charlene that now that he had gotten her back, he would never let her go. I asked him whether he would mind telling her that again in the session, and when he did so, I confirmed with Charlene that she was able to "take it in." This relationship was now a resource in Charlene's fight with the dragon and a source of healing for both partners.

A year after our last session, Charlene called to let me know how she and Jim were doing. In that time she had completed some intensive work on her trauma and had made considerable progress in treatment of her eating disorder. She had come to the conclusion, she said, that the eating problem was "simply about putting things in my mouth—which I only realized after I let myself connect with the details of the abuse." She was happy to tell me that "this marriage thing has made all the difference." She went on to say, "Every time Jim puts his arms around me—I think, we did it." Not only did she express a sense of efficacy, but she described an incident that, before the couple sessions, would have cued a long period of withdrawal and an exacerbation of her symptoms. That incident now resulted in her saying to herself, "I'm safe enough in my marriage to say to Jim, 'I think you are mad, tell me.' And he is safe enough to say, 'No, I'm not—it's just your fear coming up.' " She continued: "I still struggle, my legs still hurt, I still remember horrible things when I don't want to—but having a good marriage, it's like night and day." Calls like this remind me of why I find it so rewarding to work with survivors and their partners. We can sometimes help turn night into day.

Chapter 7

Defeating an Anxiety Disorder and Marital Distress

"I don't want a fat wife, get it?"

THE CASE OF JOAN AND DAVID

Joan and David were referred by David's individual therapist, whom he had seen over a period of 3 years. The therapist told me that David had made progress, but that the ups and downs of his relationship with his wife prevented him from really taking his life in his hands and reaching some equilibrium. David had originally entered therapy to deal with an anxiety disorder. He had had several hospitalizations, the last one being 6 years ago, and understood that many of his problems stemmed from extensive physical and emotional abuse inflicted on him by his father as a child. He refused to take any medications. He stated that he had an adverse reaction to all of them. David considered his individual therapy a success because he no longer had flashbacks or nightmares about the abuse. He also felt that he had owned his controlling behavior and tendency to strike out at his two sons, now in their 20s, and had healed the relationship with them. He told me, and his wife, Joan, agreed, that he now had considerable insight into his past and how it had affected him. His therapist told me that she had done all she could for David and that

133

his marital issues were most pertinent at present. She saw these problems as preventing David from solving his problems with his alternating hyperarousal and irritability, interspersed by numbing and periods of depression. Joan, his partner of 30 years, agreed with this synopsis and tearfully added that she would have to leave him if nothing changed and that she experienced him as "obsessed with controlling" her. David could also be considered to reflect the "covert depression" described in a recent book by Real (1997). In the terms of this book, David's need to control his wife would be considered an "addictive defense" against his own sense of vulnerability and shame arising from his trauma at the hands of his father.

It is interesting to note that David no longer experienced flashbacks and nightmares, and he did not talk about or demonstrate avoidance symptoms. The symptoms of posttraumatic stress disorder (PTSD) overlap considerably with those of other anxiety disorders, and David's problems would probably not have met the criteria for a diagnosis of full PTSD when he came for couple therapy. However, he did experience general anxiety problems and, more specifically, numbing, a restricted range of affect and detachment from others, and pronounced anger, irritability, and a desire to control others. Some recent findings suggest that these factors, in fact, best identify those suffering from PTSD (Foa & Rothbaum, 1998). Other researchers have specifically suggested that numbing and anger protect individuals from continuous anxiety when avoidance fails to do so (Riggs, Rothbaum, & Foa, 1995).

Joan and David were now in their late 50s. Joan worked at home doing accounting, and David worked as a manager in the city maintenance department. David, who was of mixed race, described his problem in the following terms. He characterized his father as the "meanest son of a bitch who ever drew breath," who used to call him "white boy" and imply that he resembled his mother and his three sisters too much. He also habitually referred to David as "Davidalina" and talked continually about how small his genitals were. At present, David said his problem was that he was "verbally mean" to his wife and was obsessed with control, especially with worrying about money and about Joan's weight. Joan, who was slim and pretty, agreed with this description and added that David had never been physically abusive to her. She said that she had grown up constantly afraid of her father and brothers, and that she had taken a knife to bed with her since the age of 10 and had never allowed anyone to hurt her physically. She had left her family home to marry David at the age of 18 and had experienced the marriage as a "happy escape" until her children came along. She had experienced serious depression after the birth of each child.

This couple scored 73 on the Dyadic Adjustment Scale (70 is typical of divorcing couples and 100 is used as the cutoff point for marital distress); David revealed a fearful-avoidant attachment style, and Joan showed an anxious-preoccupied style. When asked about their strengths as a couple, they mentioned that the first few years together were wonderful and that even now they occasionally went to a friend's cottage together and "acted like newlyweds." In the first years of their marriage, they were close, they said, and cuddled a lot. Even now, the cuddling and the sexual part of their relationship was strong. They also enjoyed having breakfast together and going out with friends.

The problem cycle in their relationship was easy to identify. David would criticize his wife and complain about her weight or her spending money. She would "clam up" and withdraw; he would then "up the ante" and become increasingly critical and denigrating until she exploded. She commented, "He hurts me to the core, so I finally try to get him to feel some of what I'm feeling." They would each withdraw for a few days, feeling very down and depressed. He would then "suck up" to her, as he put it, and for a few days things would go "okay," but then the cycle would recur. His version was, "She knifes me in the gut so I slam her." Her version was, "I buy a cushion and he hits the roof." In the first session, David moved from belligerence to near tears in a few seconds. He went from turning to me and saying, "I don't want a fat wife, get it?" to beginning to cry when describing how Joan had touched his shoulder after an argument, because it had meant so much to him. Joan also became teary during the early sessions when she spoke of the many years she spent trying to deal with David's volatility. When I asked David what happened to him as his wife expressed how tired and hopeless she felt, he stated, "Not much, I don't have much empathy—I don't feel for people." When I asked him what was happening to him as Joan spoke, he told me, "I am running my usual program, worrying about money and how much therapy is going to cost, and remembering Joan slamming me by telling our friends about how my fear of flying limits our holiday options."

In an individual session, Joan described how David told her what to wear, what aerobics class to attend, and constantly monitored and commented on her food intake. She said, "He is driving me nuts, and I am pulling away from him." She stated that she wanted to be able to run her own life and was tired of living in a house where "nothing I do is ever good enough." She spoke of living with a violent father who constantly threatened her and said that, at times, living with David felt the same. Joan said she often felt desperate, but did not want to leave David unless there was no other way. She had tried to deal with his behavior over the years by drawing boundaries. For example, she would not tell him her weight and chose her exercise options without his input. She had also left him for a week a few years ago, but had then returned. She ended the session in tears, commenting to me, "You've got to help us, we are really stuck."

David, in his individual session, spoke of how much Joan's distance hurt him and how he feared that if she got fat (as all his sisters apparently had), he would lose his arousal. Then even the sexual link between them would be broken. He spoke of his "breakdowns" and how he thought they had occurred because he had been on "overload," trying to be a "perfect" worker, father, and husband. He also spoke of his father's cruelty and how he had struggled to parent his sons and felt he had failed in this effort. He had tried to take care of his mother and sisters at home and had been on "overload" all his life. He spoke of his individual therapy and how much he felt it had helped him, although he still felt that he had "panics" and "anxiety attacks" about things like spending money. He did feel that he had learned a great deal about the trauma in his past and understood how it still colored much of how he responded to the world. For example, Joan and he had been trying to buy a car for 4 years, but he could not bear to sign any of the many deals he had made, and Joan now refused even to discuss the topic with him. He also described getting very irritable when stressed and having flashes of his father with an ugly leer on his face calling David a "eunuch." Interestingly, I noted that several times he also described himself as being unable to make decisions and so having "no balls." In this session, I needed to ascertain that there was no physical violence between David and Joan. There had been one incident very early in their relationship, but the only threat of violence in the family now came from verbal fights between David and his son, when his son came home for the weekend.

An important part of the individual session for me was personally connecting with David. Some of his responses, particularly his insistence on his right not to have a fat wife, offended me. He reminded me of the descriptions of abusive men generally given by Dutton (1995). Dutton specifically relates the vigilant need for control and coercive behaviors toward others to a history of abuse, the presence of PTSD, and insecure attachment. David also reminded me of Bowlby's (1973) point that an anger born of fear—the fear of loss—is usually the first response to perceived separation from an attachment figure. As I listened to him, I also started to understand that David was, like most of us, unable to be empathic or even respectful when either flooded with anxiety or becoming numb in order to cope with this anxiety. I was then able to remember how in the couple sessions he had, at times, been solicitous and concerned about his wife. As he spoke of having to have his finger on the pulse of every detail at home and at work in order to feel safe, I glimpsed the familiar shadow of the dragon.

STAGE 1. STABILIZATION: PROCESS STEPS

Beginning sessions were concerned with building an alliance with both partners and obtaining the information mentioned in the preceding section, as well as clearly delineating the cycle as previously described. We explored concrete instances of the steps in the cycle in the couple's daily life and as they occurred in the session. The couple called it the "C shuffle." They described it as beginning with David's contemptuous criticism, then Joan's clamming up, then more contemptuous criticism, a "catastrophic conniption fit" by Joan, then mutual clamming up, followed by David's conciliatory "sucking up" and a period of calm. The emotions that organized each step in the internal cycle were touched, named, and expanded, along with the trauma cues that potentiated them. For example, it became clear that David was always scanning the horizon for danger. If Joan wore jeans on a particular day, he might take this as a personal affront, a sign that she didn't care to look nice for him, and so he didn't matter to her. He would then criticize her dress, and she would confirm his fears by withdrawing from him. Unable to trust her love for him or their relationship, he tried to control every part of it. Parts of this cycle were explored and reframed; for example, David's lack of empathy was expanded into "shutting down" in the face of fear, in this case his fear of having failed as a spouse and so facing the loss of his wife. David began to talk more openly about his fear of being alone and of the possibility that Joan was disappointed in him. As Joan spoke of how she experienced the relationship, he began to understand viscerally how his responses affected her and how, as she put it, "He constantly drives me away from him." As in other cases, the traumatic events that had taught David particular ways of responding and the negative cycle were framed as the enemy, and the couple began to move together to face this common threat. The cycle began to slow down and the couple was able to exit from it, at least in the sessions. They did this by using humor, sharing softer feelings, or commenting on the cycle as it occurred. They began to express hope for their relationship and to find more "honeymoon times" of relaxation and sexuality together. We spoke extensively about David's being "on guard" and vigilant for threats and his longing for safety and comfort. David began to talk about how the more frequent holding that was now occurring and the signs that Joan desired him were "major safety/reassurance signals for me." Joan began to talk about her desire for more respect from David and appeared generally less depressed.

Once an alliance had been formed, the process of de-escalation and linking problematic responses in the cycle to David's anxiety and past trauma, went relatively smoothly and easily. I assumed that Stage 2 was going to be more difficult. The couple began to move into the more intense stage of therapy, in which the tasks were to restructure the emotional responses arising from past trauma and present attachment insecurities and foster positive interactions characterized by accessibility and responsiveness.

STAGE 2. RESTRUCTURING THE BOND: PROCESS STEPS AND EVENTS

In Stage 2, the goal was to continue to create new kinds of interactions that would provide a secure base and a safe haven for David, to help him explore new responses and deal with his vulnerabilities in a way that did not injure Joan and his relationship, and to foster interactions in which Joan could effectively assert her limits and needs and become less withdrawn and depressed. Joan was the more withdrawn partner and the most receptive, so we began to focus on her need to protect herself by shutting David out. Joan started by recounting an incident in which David commented that she looked fat in a new dress and she had retreated upstairs and refused to talk to him. I asked how she was feeling as she told this story.

JOAN: (*sighs—soft, low voice*) He'll never change. (*Sets her mouth, then looks down and suddenly flicks the arm of the chair with her hand.*)

THERAPIST: Your voice sounds resigned, hopeless. (*Joan nods.*) But then you set your mouth and hit the chair with your hand. [Reflecting nonverbals that may expand her dominant emotion]

JOAN: I did! (*Giggles.*)

THERAPIST: Yes, it was as if your voice was resigned—sad—but your body wanted to hit—to strike out—to fight? [Reflection and empathic inference]

JOAN: Hum. (*long pause*) Well, sometimes I feel I spend my whole life trying to please him and getting criticized. Sometimes I feel I'll just shrivel up. (*Her voice drops and becomes very soft.*) It's not right, you know.

THERAPIST: It's not right, it's not fair. It's not acceptable to be so put down, so criticized, so emotionally abused. Sometimes you feel as if you will die—you will shrivel up if it doesn't stop. [Expanding and heightening]

JOAN: (*Nods and weeps.*) I feel dreadful about myself—I get compared to 30-year-old women, and that's not right. I just withdraw to protect myself—to (*her mouth sets again and she jabs her finger at him*) get him off my back.

THERAPIST: It just hurts too much—all the put-downs, the attempts to control you. Part of you goes and curls up in your room. (*Joan weeps and nods.*) But another part, there's another part that wants to tell him, "Get off my back." [Reflecting emotions and response patterns; heightening Joan's impulse to assert herself]

JOAN: (*giggles*) Well, I guess (*looks nervously at David*) I flee instead.

THERAPIST: It's too scary to stand and fight for yourself? (*Joan tears and goes very still.*) But some part of you says you can't take it any more—don't want to take it. It's killing you. (*Joan nods.*) And the fighter part of you says, "Get off my back."

JOAN: Yes, yes (*stops crying, raises her voice, and looks at David*), or I'll find a way to leave you. I will. (*Her voice changes to a calmer and more deliberate tone.*) Yes, I will.

THERAPIST: Yes. Can you tell him, please, "Get off my back, I won't let you destroy me"? This part of you says, "I refuse to live like this," hum, is that it?

JOAN: (*Turns to David and speaks very deliberately.*) Yes, I've had it. It's enough now. It hurts too much. If I have to, well, I think I'm better off by myself. (*David goes very still and stares at the floor.*)

THERAPIST: What's happening, David? Can you hear her? (*Repeats Joan's message.*) Where are you? [Evocative inquiry]

DAVID: (*very quietly*) I hear her, but it's a long way off. I've numbed out. I'm just protecting my sanity, that's all. I think, I think I'm trying to have her prove she cares (*long silence*). It doesn't work.

THERAPIST: Can you hear her saying that you are driving her away, David? (*He nods.*) All your attempts to have her prove she cares, to test her and her caring, are driving her away.

DAVID: (*turning to the therapist*) But how can I trust her when she withdraws from me?

THERAPIST: Aha, and the less you trust, the more scared you get, and the more you watch her and test her and try to control her—and the more you drive her away.

DAVID: Right, but I'm so thin-skinned. I don't know why I don't bleed. I'm on guard all the time. (*Speaks very quietly.*) I feel small—weak.

THERAPIST: Yes, so you sort of browbeat her—then you feel bigger. (*David agrees.*) You feel more in charge, not so afraid. (*David nods and stares at the floor.*) But now Joan is saying, it's enough [Reflecting process, heightening]. Can you tell her, "When I feel small and weak, I try to be in charge of what is most important to me, you and our relationship." [Setting interactional task, choreographing a shift in his position with his wife]

After this session, Joan began to assert herself more and to withdraw less. In general, Joan's depression and negative sense of self can be viewed as a form of secondary (or vicarious) traumatic stress (STS; Barnes, 1998; Figley, 1995). Joan had been drawn into a caregiving role and, at the same time, often became the target of her partner's anger and mistrust. This combination of a sense of responsibility for the traumatized spouse, exposure to this person's anguish and painful memories, and having to deal with posttraumatic symptoms and the resulting relationship distress, render the partner extremely vulnerable to depression and anxiety. Joan often seemed caught between compassion for her spouse, fear of his hostile anger, and a desire to confront David and fight for her own needs.

It is perhaps worth commenting here on Joan's depression. Depression is very common, not only in survivors, but in their spouses as well. If we move away from a personal deficit model of depression and see depression as a signal that a person's context, his or her life situation, has gone awry, that such spouses become depressed makes perfect sense. Depression is part of Bowlby's (1969, 1981) model of separation distress and loss of closeness to an attachment figure; that is, it is an almost inevitable response to insecure attachment and marital distress. It is also a logical concomitant of the secondary traumatization that spouses such as Joan often experience. The logical response to this depression is to help the spouses change their relationship with their partners and to foster a more secure attachment that promotes healing.

As Joan became increasingly assertive and more engaged with David in the sessions and at home, David began to talk about how he had learned from his father that a man is in control in his own house. In fact, he felt out of control. He felt like a "eunuch," which is what his father used to call him. He began to talk about how he had had a vasectomy to please his wife. He, in fact, needed her caring desperately and felt really safe and reassured only when he and Joan were actually making love together. I began to focus on the fact that the more needy he felt, the more scared and helpless he felt inside. David then recounted a memory about showing his more vulnerable feelings in front of his father and being humiliated, severely beaten, and "flooded with helplessness." As mentioned previously, it is when the relationship is stabilized, the other spouse becomes available, and the survivor is invited to risk putting him- or herself in the hands of the other, that the violations of connection and traumatic images and memories become most alive and compelling. Even as David began to talk about this incident, he began to flip into rage, then into tearful longing for Joan, and finally into shame, imitating his father's voice calling him "Davidalina."

This kind of flipping between emotional states, in this case from rage to helplessness, from a sense of need and then into shame and unworthiness, is also typical at this point. The therapist slows the process, reflects, then validates and puts these responses in the context of the trauma and the present interaction. In effect, the therapist stays focused and engaged with the emotions, images, and thoughts and *offers a scaffolding to the client caught in the stream of experiencing*. The experience is then ordered and given meaning, and the emotions are regulated in the process. The therapist, in effect, helps clients engage in but also maintain a working distance (Gendlin, 1981) from difficult and potentially overwhelming emotions. We also, at the end of the session, used the frame of fearful attachment to make sense of this flipping between emotions and the impulses associated with them. At one moment, Joan seemed like the solution to all of David's fears and needs and he wanted to cling to her, then, almost at the same time, she suddenly seemed to be a source of fear and shame, and he wanted to pull away or even attack her. This paradox was paralyzing in itself. David found the frame of fearful attachment helpful and made it his own.

The images of self and the "voice" of self that arise here are also crucial. It is in the kinds of traumatic incidents that David experienced with his father, in which his vulnerability and hurt were ridiculed, that the sense of self as toxic, bad, unacceptable, and shameful is burned on the brain. These images do not seem to respond to cognitive arguments, proofs, or logic. They do seem capable of being restructured by new emotionally loaded experiences with significant others. So I asked David to hear the sneer in his own voice when he recalled his father calling him Davidalina. Did he feel that way toward his own more vulnerable self? Did he talk to his kids like that when they were vulnerable? He wept when he remembered that he had done this in the past, but said that he now had a different kind of relationship with them. However, the most important intervention was to ask Joan to share her emotions as she listened to her partner. She told him how much she respected him at this moment and how "strong" she saw him in his struggle to stay human in the face of his father's cruelty and malice. After David had gotten over his "amazement" (which took a while), he smiled broadly. Joan's acceptance of his vulnerability was an antidote to his father's contempt and offered David a new way to define himself and his vulnerability.

The couple continued to make progress. Joan firmly and calmly insisted that David trust her to manage her own body, her weight, buying groceries, and managing the house. She would not live within the narrow bounds he set. I supported her to state clear, specific limits. She said, "I'm not the enemy. It's a tea party, not a war. I'm not your child—I'm your friend. You are not my parent. I don't want to have to leave home to be grown up." David began to come to her and apologize if he had been critical and demonstrated this ability to "catch" himself "being his dad" in the session. Joan was "shocked and amazed" by this. David became much more open about confronting his relapses into the hostile mistrust modeled for him by his father.

However, he would also have "slips" and become blaming and indignant at times. At one point, he described a distressing interaction with Joan and asked me whether I agreed that he was "only 50% to blame or something like that." I replied (after having mentally checked on the strength of my alliance with him) that I thought in this instance perhaps 85% of the responsibility for the incident belonged to him and that he had probably gotten caught in his anxiety. He paused and glared at me, then burst into laughter, acknowledged his "irritability," and began to explore the triggers in the situation with Joan's help. We began to run through new response sequences in the session, in which he could perceive that a sense of "helplessness" was coming over him and be able to confide in Joan and ask for touch or reassurance. He poignantly stated, "Her touch is like a tranquillizer for me." David also went to see his mother at this point, shared some painful memories, and risked confiding in her about his struggles with his rage and his need for control.

We also began to identify clear "danger" signals that cued David's helplessness and brought up his need for control. As Wally Lamb portrays in his novel *I Know This Much Is True* (1998), certain cues trigger an urgent, compelling call for "de-fense" (as one would yell at a basketball game). David's way of dealing with his fears of loss and rejection pushed his wife away and constantly recreated the danger in the relationship, robbing him of the safe place he needed to heal. For example, if he reached for Joan and her face stayed still and she did not make immediate eye contact or smile, he would "fall off the cliff," as he described it. "The ground is gone beneath my feet. I am in free fall." Then, a second later, he would find himself thinking, "She's done it to me again—I'll show her," and he would be "lost" in the usual attempt to control and coerce. She would then see the "tyrant," not the David she loved.

More and more, David was able to experience and confide his attachment needs in the sessions. Typically, he would come to the realization that he needed Joan's nurturing, but then denigrate himself for feeling this need. So the inner sense of "I want Joan's nurturing so much" would cue the struggle with "This is weak, pathetic, unmanly." An excerpt from one of the last sessions demonstrates his struggle:

JOAN: I can't always nurture you, take care of you when you ask. I need to rest sometimes.

DAVID: I know, I'm like a sponge, but it's okay if I just know you care (*tears*).

THERAPIST: I can't believe your courage, David, in asking for caring, trusting Joan with these soft parts of you, when for so long your life depended on never doing that. (*David beams at therapist.*)

JOAN: Basically, I like it. I like to comfort him. It makes me feel good.

DAVID: And I think I have finally got around the "looking for proof she loves me and seeing her eating a muffin as proof she doesn't care" thing. I still struggle with the male thing, like, is it really okay to be soft?

JOAN: I see you struggle, but I want to tell you that it's such a relief not to have a policeman in the house. Such a relief not have to fight for my life, to fight not be taken over all the time. Because, let's be clear, at those times you become the enemy, and I won't let you destroy me. I won't let you do to me what your dad tried to do to you.

THERAPIST: Can you tell him that again, Joan? (*She does.*) Can you hear that, David?

DAVID: My God, yes, I hear it—to see it like that is hard . Yes, I hear it. That's a heavy thing. I don't want to be like him. (*Long silence—he looks at his hands.*)

THERAPIST: You don't want to be a bully like your dad, but it's so hard to risk, to show the softer side of you? (*David nods vigorously.*) Can you tell her?

DAVID: (*very quietly*) I don't want to be a bully like him, but it's very hard to admit I need you—learn to trust you, you know. It would help to know you need me too.

JOAN: David, I have been dealing with your control stuff for years to be with you. I do need you. (*David tears and reaches for Joan's hand.*) You know, the other night, when you got upset, I came and held you and told you I needed a hug too, remember? (*David nods.*) But, but, I reached past your irritation and touched you, loved you—I risked, and then you smacked me? Remember?

DAVID: Yes, I know, I know, we talked about it already. Well, what happened anyway?

JOAN: You looked down and, right out of the blue, you said to me, "Are you going to lose weight then?" And I got up and left.

THERAPIST: (*Therapist goes over the steps in this incident so that it is clear.*) So just as you were offering David the closeness you know he longs for but cannot ask for, he pulled back and became the Critic, the Boss, the Tyrant again, and the moment was lost. You moved away then? (*Joan nods emphatically.*) What happened, David, in that moment? [Therapist heightens the process of David's exit from risking to coercion.]

DAVID: Don't know, can't remember. (*Therapist leans forward and softly says, "Really?"*) Well, I guess, well, I guess I got uptight. Some part of me said, "If I just let my guard down like this and don't reserve judgment, she won't try to please me. (*Looks at therapist, who raises her eyebrows.*) Yes, yes, okay. It's so hard to let go of the control sometimes. Change is scary, you know.

THERAPIST: Yes, it is. And what I hear is that you were able to talk to Joan about this later, and you can talk about it now. It's so hard for you to trust her, isn't it? If you had stayed open and trusting when you were young, you would have died. It's a lot to learn.

DAVID: (*starting to cry*) There is a moment when I just feel so bloody helpless and all the alarms go off.

THERAPIST: (*very soft voice*) Right, and all that fear hits, the fear of putting yourself in her hands. And you stop, stand back, and judge her—push her away. Push away all the love and care that you have been longing for all these years—starving for all these years. [Heightening the attachment costs of this pattern, as well as the attachment longings]

DAVID: That's right. (*Weeps long and hard; Joan leans forward and strokes his knee.*)

After this session, David and Joan made great progress. They went on a trip for their anniversary, and Joan said that she felt they recaptured the joy they had had when they were first married. David commented, "If I can just take the risk and let her in, she takes all the hurt out of me." David also talked about a long conversation with a family friend in which they discussed what being a man was about and shared different images of what it meant to be strong. David gathered from this friend that he did act in ways that reminded this friend of David's father at times, and concluded, "I'm only like him when my fear is controlling me. I don't want to be a bully like him." He was able to turn to Joan and say, "I want to trust you. Can you help me? It's one step at a time." Her soft smile and her touch told him the answer to his question.

David was right, it was one step at a time, and by the next time they came for a session, there had been a serious episode when David had relapsed into, as Joan put it, "his policing and controlling act." This time, however, with very little help from me, Joan really asserted herself and insisted that if he could not respect her, she would have to leave. David was then able to look again at his anxiety and how the ways he managed it trapped them both in despair, and apologized to his wife. David opened one of the last sessions with an observation in perfect contrast to his opening remarks in the first session. In the first session he had begun with "I don't want a fat wife." In this session, after general niceties about how they were doing, he looked at his wife and said, "You look absolutely ravishing today," and then burst into tears. When we explored this a little, he was able to say that his tears were about his belief that when Joan dressed well and showed she cared about her weight, he took this as evidence that she loved him and cared about how he saw her, and so the relationship was safe. Joan took the compliment, but then was able to tell David that she did not want to look good all the time just to reassure him. She didn't want to dress a certain way in order to show David that she cared about his approval. In the following dialogue, taken from this session, it may be possible to detect not just a contrast with beginning sessions, but some markers of more secure attachment that indicate the end of Stage 2 of EFT. The markers I noticed were that the couple could detach from their negative cycle and confront each other with humor; that they could, as is typical of secure partners, meta-communicate; that both were more assertive and able to state their needs clearly; and that they could emotionally engage and comfort and reassure each other.

DAVID: I get stuck in this silly thing, where if she doesn't care what she looks like—if she wears that old yellow nightgown (*grimacing*), then I think she doesn't care about me. And then I get all freaked out. I'm really working hard at this, you know. I shut my mouth when she gets into that nightgown.

JOAN: (*giggling*) Well, I feel more able to say what I think, and I want to be in that old nightgown sometimes, so . . . (*Smiles at David and shrugs; David smiles back.*)

THERAPIST: David, how do you feel when Joan says this? What's it like for you when she stands up to you and tells you that you have to learn to risk and trust? She won't always do what reassures you and proves her love.

DAVID: It's okay—yeah, I like it. I'm letting go of the reins more. I like her saying what she wants. I like it better than us being distant for days. (*Joan nods.*)

THERAPIST: You feel better too, Joan?

JOAN: Oh yes. I can say stuff now and he can hear it. Like the other day, he got tense 'cause I was eating chocolates (*David nods and smiles*), and I told him, we get stuck here. I said, this is where you push me away by being bossy. You let me look after me, and you just get on with your own life. His being a policeman just drives a wedge between us.

THERAPIST: It feels good, strong, to say to David, "You look after your own life and leave me to deal with mine"? (*Joan nods and beams at therapist.*)

DAVID: She's right, too. And because that's happening we can talk more and play more—like throwing shirts at each other the other night. (*Both David and Joan dissolve into laughter.*)

THERAPIST: So you can catch yourself before you step into the policeman role, and Joan can also stop you and insist you step to the side. (*David agrees.*) And can you also go to her when your anxiety is rising and tell her, so she can help you with it? Can you pull her close when you need her help to calm down?

DAVID: Sometimes. (*Turns to Joan.*) Do I, dear? (*Joan mentions several instances, during the weeks since the therapist had last seen them, when David had done this.*)

JOAN: And you are much more generous, giving praise and saying I look nice. You're working hard in lots of ways. (*To the therapist*) He even went out and bought a stereo, just like that, after all this time—said it helped his anxiety. (*Therapist expresses amazement. David giggles.*) The other day, walking along the street, in public, he got all critical with me, and I just said, "Stop being such a jackass." And he did!

THERAPIST: Even when David slips into being a policeman, you don't get so intimidated and withdraw into getting depressed? You don't let David's slips into bossiness depress you anymore?

JOAN: Right. I don't get into the "I will never please him" thing. Sometimes I want to be in my old snuggly yellow nightgown.

THERAPIST: You are doing really well together. I don't think you need me anymore.

DAVID: We were talking about that on the way here, It's a bit scary, though. This stuff helped a lot.

THERAPIST: Do you know what helped most, David?

DAVID: Well, we got to see the big picture—not so caught in details and our own knee-jerk reactions. And then, the way you listened—I got that I wasn't crazy or hopeless after all. Even when you gave me a hard time, confronted me, I felt important in here and that you cared about me.

JOAN: I liked the way you zeroed in—on emotions and stuff. You were active, but you felt safe to me. I think we have come a long way.

DAVID: And I'm not even going to take the stereo back later. (*All three laugh.*)

The rest of the final sessions were taken up with the Stage 3 tasks of integration, such as formulating a narrative of the change process and the victories the couple had experienced in this process. Part of the process involved each partner explicitly describing how his or her sense of self changed when they were able to feel secure together and support each other. We also engaged in problem solving as to how they planned to deal with relapses into the criticism–withdrawal pattern in the future. At the end of therapy this couple scored 106 on the Dyadic Adjustment Scale (over 100 is considered nondistressed). The sessions ended with the couple being able to initiate and maintain bonding sequences of caring and comfort and to contain and repair the negative interactions that left them both isolated and hurting. David was able to stop "setting fire to the house I live in." I complimented them both on their courage and how, for both of them, fighting for their relationship had meant staring down 50 years of fear. I wished for them that they might drive into the sunset, in a new car. David said the car decision might take a little while.

This case illustrates the long-term effects of complex PTSD and how such effects undermine the secure attachment required for healing. Cases of this kind also illustrate that, because the self is defined in relation to others, shifting one's position in a relationship with an attachment figure is a powerful route to defining oneself differently. Fonagy and Target (1997) point out that when individuals grow up traumatized and without any secure attachment figures, they miss out on the mirroring that fosters an ability to reflect on the self and create a coherent state of mind about the self. Secure attachment, and the capacity to regulate and process emotions that comes with it, strengthens the ability to stand back and reflect on oneself and one's behavior, intentions, and mental states, which, in turn, promotes individual transformations and the renewal of intimate bonds.

Chapter 8

The Trauma of Physical Illness

"I can face dying. But I don't want to die alone."

The traditional marriage vows promise steadfastness "in sickness and in health." The significance of this promise is emphasized by a substantial body of research that links mortality and many forms of physical and mental "dis-ease" to isolation. Social isolation is a major risk factor for cardiovascular disease, for example (Krantz, Contrada, Hill, & Friedler, 1988). Isolation also exacerbates stressful events and chronic stress and is associated with the down-regulation of immune function (Kiecolt-Glaser & Glaser, 1995), as are divorce and bereavement. In general, emotions seem to have direct effects on "stress" hormones and they, in turn, can modulate immune function. Negative emotions are not then just "in the head." As the trauma literature has always suggested, they can and do have a real negative impact on how the body functions. Stress, isolation, and pain delay the healing of wounds and surgical recovery (Kiecolt-Glaser, Page, Marucha, MacCallum, & Glaser, 1998). In general, the adverse health outcomes associated with lack of social support appear to be comparable to those associated with smoking (House et al., 1988). Indirect effects may

---

This case was first reported in Johnson (1999). Copyright by The Guilford Press. Adapted by permission.

increase the risk; for example, depression after a heart attack has a major impact on recovery (Carney et al., 1988), and we know that marital distress has robust links with depression.

We can even specify negative events in a relationship that appear to affect health. Negative emotional states orient people to respond to proximal immediate events (Frijda, 1986) and can interfere with planning for the future. In general, there is increasing evidence that there are many ways in which negative emotions can impact physical and mental health (Salovey, Rothman, Deitweiler, & Steward, 2000). Negative interactions, such as demand–withdraw, can lead to significant immune system down-regulation and cardiovascular reactivity (Kiecolt-Glasser et al., 1993). Hostility and criticism by attachment figures appear to predict relapse into mental health problems such as depression (Hooley, 1990) Criticism and distancing by a spouse also appear to elicit more maladaptive coping strategies from women who are coping with chronic illness (Manne & Zautra, 1989). When spouses are critical of them, symptoms of traumatic stress in cancer patients, such as intrusive thoughts, are also more distressing (Manne, 1999).

On the other hand, we know that the presence of a positive, close relationship is one of the best predictors of physical and mental health and longevity (Burman & Margolin, 1992; Schmaling & Sher, 2000). As King Solomon suggests in Proverbs 17, "A merry heart doeth good like a medicine." More specifically, heart patients and those with chronic pain who have supportive spouses seem to take less pain medication, to recover more quickly, and to be rehospitalized less often (Jamison & Virts, 1990; Kulik & Mahler, 1989). As Rolland (1994) suggests, health problems are like other life challenges; they can bring couples together and promote the growth of a relationship, or they can drive partners apart. However, there is very little literature on the specific interventions for couples dealing with illness and even less on interventions for couples for whom traumatic experience is part of that illness. Cognitive-behavioral approaches advocate the use of education, communication, and problem-solving skills (Halford, Scott, & Smythe, 2000; Schmaling, & Sher, 1997) for couples facing serious illness. Other systemic interventions focus on life cycle issues (Rolland, 1999). Here, the focus is on the quality of the attachment and emotional engagement between spouses. Among the various possible kinds of support, it is emotional support from partners that is most frequently desired by patients with illnesses such as cancer. Emotional support is also rated as being the most helpful type of support and having the strongest links with long-term adjustment (Helgeson & Cohen, 1996). The quality of the attachment between spouses seems to have an effect even beyond the grave. Even when illness results in the death of a partner, insecure attachment is associated with less ability to handle grief and more traumatic grief symptoms (van Doorn, Kasl, Berry, Jacobs, & Prigerson, 1998).

A number of people who face serious illness also meet the criteria for an anxiety disorder, such as posttraumatic stress disorder (PTSD). Up to 10% of breast cancer patients, for example, meet the criteria for PTSD (Cordova et al., 1995) and may continue to meet those criteria for many years after diagnosis. In my experience, this is more likely to occur if the patient and his or her partner were distressed in their relationship when the illness occurred, and if the partner has significant difficulty in coping with the illness of the patient. A serious illness such as cancer often induces emotional changes in both partners, including heightened uncertainty and vulnerability, and a redefinition of life goals and priorities.

THE CASE OF LEN AND CLARA

Len and Clara were an older couple coping with lung cancer and the traumatic stress this involved, a life transition into retirement, and a distressed relationship.

The individual therapist who had seen Clara for more than a year reported that Clara suffered from intrusive thoughts, flashbacks of her cancer diagnosis and treatment, inability to sleep, and general hyperarousal and irritation. This therapist diagnosed the condition as partial PTSD with significant depression. Clara had made progress; however, her improvement was not stable and her depression was not abating. The therapist recognized that the longstanding distress in the relationship between Clara and Len was maintaining Clara's problems, and, in fact, the relationship problems appeared to be multiplying and Clara had began to talk of leaving Len. At this point Len's individual therapist, who was treating him for clinical depression, consulted with Clara's therapist, and together they decided that what was really needed was couple therapy. Len's therapist suggested that Clara's cancer and the course of her treatment had been exceedingly difficult for Len, coming as they did just as he was entering retirement and counting on the relationship with his wife to help him with that process. When I first saw the couple, it was clear to me that Len was indeed experiencing a significant level of secondary traumatization.

Clara, a small, pretty lady in her 60s, had been married to Len, her tall, gangly partner, for 40 years. While he lounged in his chair and spoke in a slow drawl (reminding me of John Wayne), she sat, alert and tight-lipped, on the edge of her chair. They told me with pride that they had three children, all of whom had left home, and two grandchildren. Len was a high-profile politician who was, as mentioned earlier, being treated for a serious depression. This depression had developed after Len had finally decided to retire because of his arthritis. Clara had undergone extensive treatment for lung cancer the year before. She told me in a steady voice that she felt that she had beaten the disease, but that there was a very high risk of recurrence and this was something she had spoken about with her individual therapist.

Clara described the problem in her relationship with Len as "constant bickering" and said that unless something changed, she was going to leave Len and "find some peace." She said that if her life was not to be long, it could at least be peaceful. Clara referred to a particular past episode a number of times. At one point, she said, Len had become very stressed and overwhelmed in his job and had pressured her to help run his office. Clara said, passionately, "I hated this job. I told him again and again that I had to stop. I told him the job was killing me." She described how he had minimized her distress at the time, and indeed he continued to do so in the session. He told her that she was exaggerating, turning to me and telling me that she "really didn't mind that much." As he smiled and informed me that his wife would "calm down in a minute," she spat out angrily that he had pressured her to keep on running the office for a year, even though she had been complaining of feeling ill and depressed, until she had finally been diagnosed with cancer. His unwillingness to listen to her was then associated with the occurrence of a life-threatening illness. This continued to be a reality for Clara, who spoke about how ill she felt when they would fight and how she feared that her distress with Len would spark a recurrence of her cancer, or at the very least undermine her ability to fight such a recurrence.

Len and Clara played out the dominant cycle in their relationship while discussing this incident. She attacked him, saying, "You discounted me and only took care of yourself, and I hate you for this." He completely dismissed her statement, responding with, "It wasn't that bad, and you don't hate me. And I took care of you when you were really ill, after your big operation." As Len defended himself in a calm, reasoning manner, Clara became increasingly enraged. "I'm tired of being told how I feel and who I am," she said. "This has gone on for 15 years, and now I'm on the point of leaving." Len's manner immediately changed when she said this. He went silent and very still. He then turned to me and began to tell a rambling, detailed story designed to prove his point, that Clara hadn't been very upset about working in his office. Clara looked as though she was going to explode and then sighed and told me in a quiet, hopeless tone, "He buries me in words." She commented that this kind of interaction occurred frequently at home and that the stress it created "is going to make me sick again." She then described images of the terror and pain involved in her cancer treatment and how these would recur when she felt discounted by Len. As she said this, he furrowed his brow and looked really upset for the first time in the session.

The specific episodes that Clara described could be labeled as an attachment injury or relationship trauma (Johnson et al., 2001) that compounded the traumatic stressors in this couple's life. Clara had expressed her exhaustion and distress, and Len had not responded. He had discounted her pain and remained inaccessible, both in the past and in the current dialogue. Underlying many such attachment injuries, which often continue to define the relationship long after the injurious event, is an potent experience of danger or physical threat in which the survivor's partner was perceived as failing to provide caring and protection. These relationship traumas are discussed in more detail in Chapter 10.

Clara and Len presented a classic cycle of complain/attack versus stonewall/defend. In this case, Len was withdrawn and clinically depressed. In retirement, he was facing a significant life transition, which he experienced as an enormous loss, and he also faced the loss of his wife to illness or divorce. In the past, Clara had usually initiated closeness, but she had now put up a "wall." Len commented that he would try to cuddle her in the mornings in bed, but he felt "pushed away." Again and again he would comment to me, "She exaggerates; she gets wild-eyed over nothing." Clara acknowledged that Len had taken care of her after her cancer surgery and during particular crises in her treatment, but then she wagged her finger at him, saying, "Mostly though, through the years, you've taught me to be alone. You've put your career first." Illness was very present in this relationship. Clara's sister had recently died of cancer, her daughter was chronically ill, and the specter of a possible return of Clara's cancer was always near. She said, with tears in her eyes, "If I have a shortened life to live, I'm determined not to live it in a box, with him sitting on the lid. I'm tired of trying to get through to him. It makes me ill."

STAGE 1. STABILIZATION: PROCESS STEPS AND KEY EVENTS

After the initial sessions and the building of an alliance, the couple and I articulated the interactional cycle described earlier, putting each person's responses in the context of the other's behavior. The couple were framed as victims of this cycle of angry complaint and rationalizing defense. They were also described as both facing traumatic changes and losses. Len responded to his sense of helplessness by "numbing" and denial, whereas Clara became hyperaroused and agitated. The interactional cycle had robbed them of the comfort and closeness they had experienced earlier in their relationship, which had sustained them through previous crises. They told their story of the evolution of the relationship. Clara said that for many years she "had allowed him to define reality," and Len admitted that he had been "rather authoritarian." She felt "bullied by his impenetrable rationalizing." He spoke of the need to persuade her to "dampen down her feelings about a few isolated negative incidents." Past events in the couple's personal histories and in the history of the relationship were pursued only if they were directly relevant to present attachment issues, problematic interactions, and trauma symptoms. Len pointed out that in his career, there were many times when it was very important for him to stay cool and calm and to rationalize people's complaints. I used this disclosure to validate that this style of coping had often been useful for him. We were then able to talk about how, here, it simply seemed to make his wife more angry and increase the distance between them. It also left them both isolated when their worse fears came over them. Clara agreed and spoke of flashbacks from her experience with cancer and how debilitating they were, especially when she was unable to turn to Len for support.

The couple then moved to exploring the emotions underlying their interactional positions. Len began to talk about his hurt at being "shut out" by Clara and by her threats to leave him. I focused on his voice and facial expression, rather than his words, and slowly helped him to formulate the realization that he was "sad" and "in shock." Gradually, he was able to talk about his fear of losing Clara, whether through her angry distancing, her leaving the relationship, or a recurrence of her illness. We began to talk about how this fear paralyzed him. Clara spoke of her sense of having no impact on Len, no way of getting him to acknowledge her hurt and desperateness, and so alternating between rage and helplessness. I helped Len to articulate that the loss of his career, in which he felt affirmed and competent, had left him feeling vulnerable and sensitive to Clara's criticism. She was able to talk of how she felt abandoned and disqualified by his "denials and discounts," and now by his withdrawal into depression. I described both of them as isolated and vulnerable and as having lost a sense of control over their lives and their relationship.

The experience and expression of the emotions implicit in the interactional cycle began to expand the dialogue, and moments of engagement began to occur. For example, when Clara talked openly of her cancer, Len was able to directly express his fear of losing her. She was touched by this expression. She commented to him, "I never knew you were that worried. Maybe you're just trying to calm yourself down with all that rationalizing. I thought you were just trying to bully me." Then she reached over and laid her hand on his arm.

I then set interactional tasks based on these emotional responses, which promoted the de-escalation of the problem cycle and the beginning of emotional engagement. For example, I asked Len to talk to Clara about how he had lost his sense of power and competence when he retired and now also felt ashamed that he had found this so difficult to deal with. Together, we articulated that his "job" now was to take care of Clara and that he didn't know how to do it. "In fact," he said, "I'm blowing it. I'm failing." His response to this sense of failure was to feel hopeless and then withdraw. Clara began to view his withdrawal in terms of how much impact she had, rather than how little. He became less distant and self-protective, and she became less angry and blaming. At this point, the relationship became more stable and they were able to they talk about the cycle and their "sensitivities" as the problem. They were kinder to each other. They validated each other's courage in facing the "dragons" they were facing and began to see a way to face them together.

The goal at this point in therapy is for first one partner and then the other to begin to formulate and express attachment-related affect in a way that fosters acceptance from the other and rapidly reorganizes attachment behaviors. These changes then create a safe haven from which to face the dragon.

STAGE 2. RESTRUCTURING THE BOND

In Session 6, Len began to express, with much weeping, how terrified he was of Clara's anger and of hearing her say that he had failed her. Her illness, his retirement, and his own depression had all intensified his awareness of how much he needed her. As we explored what happened to him when he got the message that he was disappointing her, he was able to describe the panic that preceded his attempts to "cool down" her anger. He was then able to move into a more engaged position and ask her to stop threatening to leave and give him a chance to show her he cared. He described his experience of her rage and how he "fled into denying what was happening." He asked her to begin to control her rage, so that he could, as he put it, "learn to take care of her and become good at this new job."

Len's re-engagement allowed Clara to move into formulating her own sense of helplessness when he discounted her experience and her need for his validation and comfort. She moved, in terms of her interactional position, from a blaming stance to expressing her fear of having her pain denied and therefore being abandoned. She said to him, "It's too scary for me to count on you when you don't even seem to see or hear me." Both partners became much more available and responsive to each other and began to be able to comfort each other. They also formulated a clear narrative of how they had neglected their relationship, so that when the trauma of cancer occurred, they were unable to support each other. The cancer also came at a time when Len was facing a significant life transition, which made his wife's struggle with cancer even more overwhelming for him.

A new cycle of closeness and comfort began to emerge, and this couple was able to create pragmatic solutions to old issues, such as Len's occasional inebriation and its effect on Clara. She was able to tell him that she needed him to "be with" her, rather than against her or distant from her, and to elaborate on the times when she was most vulnerable and her need for him was most pressing. By the end of 12 sessions, this couple's interactional patterns had changed. They were able to curtail the problem cycle when it occurred and to respond to each other in a manner that initiated new cycles of closeness and confiding. Each partner's characterizations of their relationship and the other partner had changed. Clara saw her husband as overwhelmed and afraid, rather than as a bully. He saw her as desperate for his validation and caring, rather than as hysterical and hostile. Each partner's sense of self had also expanded. For example, Len was able to accept his vulnerability and feel a sense of competence in dealing with his affect and responding to his wife's needs. As a result, he became less depressed. By the end of therapy, their emotional experience was formulated differently. They were able to accept their own emotions and express them in a way that pulled them closer. They were also able to use the relationship to regulate distress and trauma symptoms, such as panic attacks about the recurrence of Clara's illness.

DEALING WITH RELAPSE

Traumatized couples are dealing with such compelling emotions and enormous existential issues that they are more likely than nontraumatized partners to experience relapses during the course of therapy. Once the therapist learns to be aware of this possibility, he or she becomes better at helping a couple deal with a relapse, learn from it, and begin moving forward again. It is only in the movies that heroes face dragons by marching steadfastly toward them. Most of us take two or three steps back before we finally grapple with the beast.

In Session 11 with Len and Clara, a relapse began to occur.

LEN: The relationship is better. I don't spend near as much energy dodging her rage. She's less angry. (*Smiles at Clara.*)

CLARA: (*Smiles back at Len.*) Well, you hear me more, and you're less depressed and withdrawn, so it's less lonely for me. But (*turning to therapist, her voice becoming higher and more clipped*) I have to be sure that he really gets this, that he can keep on doing this.

LEN: (*Studies the nails on his right hand and says slowly*) I'm not stupid. I understand more than you give me credit for. (*Looks out the window.*)

CLARA: (*Her voice now goes up a decibel, and she moves to the edge of her seat.*) Well, when you have more than one drink, you get really pushy and loud. Then on Saturday you got all mopey and distant.

LEN: (*very slowly, still looking out the window*) I got a little pushy, and I got a little down (*long pause*), but I wasn't that bad. (*Tears and looks away.*)

THERAPIST: What's happening for you now, Len? (*He mutters that he's fine.*) What's it like for you when Clara says she sees you as being easier for her to get close to, to contact, and then she adds a "but"?

LEN: I don't like it. It's hard. (*Looks directly at Clara, but she stares at her hand. He begins to weep.*)

THERAPIST: Aha. It's hard. And some part of you even feels like weeping, is that right?

LEN: (*pause; focusing on therapist and rubbing his eyes*) No, not weeping. No, it's just my eyes watering (*long pause*). Well, okay, it's like she's accusing me again, and that's scary.

THERAPIST: Right. And that's part of the cycle you both get trapped in.

LEN: Right (*long silence and then a deep sigh*). Maybe I can't make it.

CLARA: (*Looking up at Len, her voice is soft, and she sits back in her chair.*) I'm trying to give you a chance. We've had some really good days. (*Her lips tighten again; she smoothes her skirt with her hand.*) But then, I gave you the recipe, I suggested no alcohol and . . .

THERAPIST: (*deciding to stay with Len and help him stay engaged; using a soft voice*) You're disappointed that she is doubting you?

LEN: Yeah, she starts to accuse me (*turning to Clara*). I can read recipes, but . . . (*Tears and wrings his hands.*)

THERAPIST: What happened on Saturday afternoon, Len, before you had a few drinks?

LEN: I got into a . . . (*searching for the right words, then speaking emphatically and deliberately*) a massive internal flap.

THERAPIST: A massive internal flap—can you help me understand? Is being in a flap like being frantic?

LEN: Yeah. She was talking about the drinking, and I was already uneasy, but then, but then . . . (*Len's voice cracks and he squirms in his chair*) she went in the study and read the medical books my brother gave me. (*He weeps.*)

CLARA: (*turning to the therapist and speaking in a very calm tone*) I went and read about my kind of cancer, and it wasn't good. It said that, basically, recurrence is just a matter of time.

LEN: And she still has that pain. (*Puts his hands over his eyes.*)

CLARA: (*leaning toward Len and speaking calmly*) But we knew that, really.

THERAPIST: You were able to read the book and look at that with some calmness, Clara? (Clara nods). But for you, Len, anticipating that Clara is about to be disappointed with you or angry at you was difficult—that's still difficult—but then knowing that she had read that book, the book you had already read, yes? (*Len nods and his eyes widen, indicating that therapist is on track here.*) That bought on a massive internal flap, a panic, for you, yes?

LEN: Yes. (*He weeps.*) I want to make her happy. I try. Her anger scares me. She talks of leaving, and we've got better at handling that, but then, then she talked about this recurrence thing and life being short. (*His voice trails off.*)

THERAPIST: And you start to feel helpless (*Len nods*), as though you can't make her happy—at least that's what came up on Saturday afternoon—and you fear that you might loose her, she might leave, by getting mad enough at you, or by getting sick again. Is that it? [Reflecting and heightening panic and fear of loss]

LEN: Yes. (*He weeps.*) She used to say the fights we had were killing her. Things have improved a lot, but . . . Saturday . . .

CLARA: (*Now looks concerned and leans toward Len. She sees his distress. She looks much more concerned than she was the first time she went through the process of Len's expressing and owning his hurts and fears.*) I know I have said that you're not listening and discounting me kills me, but . . .

THERAPIST: (*to Len*) On Saturday afternoon all your fears of not being able to hold onto Clara, of not being able to keep her, keep her happy and with you, of losing her, came up again, yes? (*Len nods emphatically.*) You even heard her say that the relationship was hurting her, making her sick, and you got frantic.

LEN: That's it. (*He weeps and wipes the tears away.*) It's terrifying. I get totally paralyzed, I do.

THERAPIST: And that's the massive internal flap that has you minimizing and trying to persuade Clara that she doesn't hurt, that everything is fine. Finally, when that doesn't work, you feel beaten and you withdraw into your despair, that's what it's all about? (*Thera-*

pist summarizes the inner panic that primes Len's despair and his withdrawal.)

LEN: Right, I get all scared. I hover around, trying to be optimistic, and she feels discounted.

CLARA: (*looking surprised*) But you were always so separate, so into your work. I never felt you even needed me.

THERAPIST: It's a little strange for you to hear his fear, isn't it? To see how much he needs you, how afraid he is of hurting or disappointing you?

CLARA: (*long pause, staring at Len*) I guess so . . . so, so, you're afraid. (*Len nods and tears.*)

THERAPIST: Maybe he's even more afraid of fighting the cancer again than you are?

CLARA: (*again in a surprised tone*) Oh . . . oh, well, I guess so . . . yes, maybe he is.

THERAPIST: His massive internal flap pulls him into trying to make everything smooth, better. He tries to make your hurts smaller, but then you get even more hurt and angry, and he gets defeated and depressed. You're so precious to him—is that okay, Len? (*Len nods.*) He goes into a panic.

Len's minimizing and discounting are framed in an attachment context. All these formulations of underlying feelings and empathic inferences have been used before. They are now applied specifically in the context of Clara's possible relapse and his fear of that happening.

CLARA: Oh. . . . (*She turns to Len.*) Is that it?

LEN: (*in a much more relaxed tone*) That's about it. When you get in a hissy fit and say you're leaving, I just can't handle that. And then you tell me that the way I am with you will bring back the cancer . . . I just freeze up.

CLARA: (*putting her hands up to her face*) Oh dear, maybe I shouldn't do that.

LEN: (*leaning toward Clara*) It would help. I'm trying. I think I'm doing better. I wasn't good at listening in the past. I can't handle being afraid of losing you and then hearing that I'm making you sick. I want to be with you, not hurt you.

THERAPIST: (*softly*) What happens for you as you see his fear, Clara?

CLARA: Well, I guess . . . it all seems different. It puts things in a different light.

THERAPIST: Aha. Maybe it's his fear that he is trying to control when he plays down your feelings and withdraws.

CLARA: Right, and I always saw it as his trying to control me!

LEN: (*Smiles at Clara and then at therapist; he's John Wayne again.*) I wouldn't dare. (*He laughs.*)

THERAPIST: Len, can you help Clara see more? Can you help her understand how much you want to protect and hold her, how afraid you are when the shadow of her leaving, through anger or getting ill, looms?

I then drew the session to a close on the theme of how fear isolated them from each other. All of the themes explored in this session had been touched on before, and the couple had already changed their problem cycle and initiated a more positive bond. They had completed Stage 2 of therapy. However, here all of these themes came together and could be addressed in an integrated fashion that prevented relapse, consolidated his engagement and her softening, and explicitly brought the issue of cancer into the interaction. This session was then a watershed between Stage 2 and Stage 3 of therapy. The next session covered all the Stage 3 processes and was the last. The couple came in and reported that they had talked for hours together about Clara's need to be seen by Len and to depend on his responsiveness, and about his fears of failing her and losing her. This process was a repeat and an elaboration of the initial process of Len's reengagement that had occurred in earlier sessions. Clara was able to respond here because she had already expressed her needs in a previous session and experienced his comfort and caring.

They also reported that they had talked openly during the previous week of the possibility of Clara's death and experienced being much closer to each other. She stated that she realized that because they were closer, she felt "no panic" about the idea of a recurrence of her illness. She said to me in a quiet voice, "If it happens, we will face it together." The couple had also been able to talk together and formulate pragmatic plans and coping strategies to deal with such a recurrence. They were able to use their relationship as a safe haven and a secure base in dealing constructively with the trauma of cancer.

Many things happened in these last two sessions in regard to the individual partners, relationship definition, and existential realities. Specifically, this session touched on Len's depression and adjustment to retirement, the nature of the couple's attachment and marital satisfaction, and their ability to cope with the traumatic stressors of cancer and the possibility of a recurrence of Clara's illness and her possible death.

To further clarify the process of change, it may be useful to look at key moments in Clara's softening and allowing herself to be vulnerable so that she could begin to trust her partner, and how these moments redefined the relationship:

- In Session 2, Clara formulated the emotions underlying her critical, angry stance in terms of helplessness. She said, "I can't get through to him. I hurl myself at this mountain. He just defines me away. He says I don't hurt."
- In the Stage 2 softening process, in Session 6, Clara was able to tell Len, "I get desperate when you discount me. It's as though I don't exist. It's as though I've died already. It's like when I said I felt ill before the cancer diagnosis, you said I was fine, but I was dying." (She wept.) "I can't reach you."
- In Session 8, this process evolved into Clara's stating with quiet intensity her fear of abandonment and her need for comfort. She said, "I'm afraid of the cancer coming back, but I'm more afraid of being alone. I need you to see me and hold me. Hold me so I'm not so afraid. Please don't leave me all alone." She got up and held onto Len.

When these moments occurred:

1. Clara focused on and expressed vulnerability rather than anger. She was then able to formulate her needs. She was also able to express them in a way that made it easier for Len to respond. It is when we are experiencing intense emotion that we find it easiest to formulate our most pressing needs and concerns. Emotion carries with it a clear message about what matters most to us.

2. Clara's expression of vulnerability constituted a less dominant, more affiliative stance toward Len. Emotion is an action tendency; as Clara experienced her fear and longing, she reached for Len and asked for comfort. In doing so, she changed her interactional position. She was no longer simply the critical accuser.

3. As Clara expressed her fears and hurts, Len saw her differently. She was less dangerous. She was therefore easier for him to respond to. The expression of "new" emotion pulls for a "new" response from the spouse and so reorganizes the interaction, creating a shift from the problem cycle.

4. Len was able to touch his sense of failure in this process and have it evolve into a new sense of how essential and irreplaceable he was to his wife. As interactions expand, so does each partner's sense of self. Both partners see themselves as more able to control their relationship and deal with their emotions. Intense emotions are a direct route into our core cognitions about who we are.

5. New emotions structured new steps in Len and Clara's dance. A new cycle of confiding and responsiveness began. Such a new cycle of trust and confiding creates a more positive relationship and tends to be self-reinforcing.

6. Len and Clara's new cycle was not just a new set of behaviors replacing a destructive cycle. It was a cycle that addressed inherent attachment needs. It redefined the relationship as a place of safety and comfort. This, then, influenced both partners' resilience in the face of illness, loss, and death.

Chapter 9

Couple Therapy
with Combat Veterans

"I need you to be my ears . . . my safety."

THE CASE OF ROBERT AND ELIZABETH

This chapter deals with a course of marital therapy involving combat-related posttraumatic stress disorder (PTSD). The husband had been in Vietnam for two tours of duty. Research suggests that social support plays a key role in coping with combat stress (Keane, Scott, Chavoya, Lamparski, & Fairbank, 1985; Solomon, Waysman, & Mikulincer, 1990; Solomon, Mikulincer, & Habershaim, 1990). It is also clear that PTSD has a "substantial negative impact not only on the veterans' own lives, but also on the lives of spouses, children and others living with such veterans" (Kulka et al., 1990, p. 28). Depression and substance abuse associated with combat stress are also often implicated in veterans' marital difficulties. Rob and Elizabeth were married partners in their late 40s at the time of therapy. The first tour of duty for Rob, a Canadian Vietnam veteran, was very early in the war, and he had been involved in an explosion of a land mine. In this incident, he sustained a traumatic injury to his spine. Luckily for him, when the enemy came upon him, he was able to feign death, and they passed him by after

---

Lyn Williams Keeler was the therapist in this case and coauthor of this chapter.

164

putting a bullet into the head of his injured buddy. He was shipped out of Vietnam to recover from his wounds.

Driven by a desire to prove he could stand in combat, he returned a couple of years later to do a second tour as a member of the military police unit stationed in Saigon. At the time he had gone to Vietnam for his first tour of duty, he was an idealistic and adventurous youth who wanted to save the world from communism. There was little evidence of traumatic experience in Rob's background before Vietnam; however, during his first tour he saw many things that clearly continued to haunt him. It is clear that war zone stress, in and of itself, makes a substantial contribution to the development of PTSD in veterans, independent of a broad range of potential predisposing factors (Fontana, Rosenheck, & Brett, 1992; King, King, Foy, & Gudanowski, 1996; Kulka et al., 1990). In the course of couple therapy, images of Rob's Vietnam experience often emerged as the source of his struggle with fear and issues of personal effectiveness and protectiveness.

When working with couples, one of whom is a combat veteran, it is not unusual to find that the other partner is someone who prefers a caretaking role. This was certainly true of Elizabeth. She had been brought up in a family in which she had been fairly well protected from life, but she had to abide by the rules her mother set out as appropriate and proper for a young girl. She was a nurse by profession and was already raising two children on her own when she met Rob. Rob had also been married before, and he had had several stormy, short-term relationships following the end of his first marriage. This pattern too is not unusual for Vietnam veterans, whose relationship history often seems to reflect a fearful-avoidant style of attachment whereby they pursue relationships but then cannot deal with the anxieties of depending on their partners. They then have problems with trust and maintaining closeness. As discussed in Chapter 2, PTSD, with its alternating hyperarousal and numbing, wreaks havoc with the creation and maintenance of a secure attachment. The lack of secure attachment then tends to exacerbate and maintain the symptoms of PTSD. Research suggests that the degree of distress in veterans' relationships is associated particularly with the symptoms of emotional numbing (Riggs et al., 1998) and motional numbing seems to be even more strongly related to relationship quality than effortful avoidance symptoms.

Rob and Elizabeth were referred to couple therapy by a colleague, who had been working with Rob on an adequate assessment of his PTSD. In fact, on the Clinician Administered PTSD Scale, Rob had scored 108 on the three symptom criteria. Because a score of 70 is generally considered to indicate moderate PTSD, this score indicated fairly severe PTSD. Rob himself informed the therapist in the early sessions that he was the "sick" one who deserved most of the therapeutic attention and focus, because he lived every day with the debilitating symptoms of PTSD. Rob refused to fill out the Dyadic Adjustment Scale to assess the distress in his marriage, and his wife complied with his wishes and also declined to complete this measure.

The only reason Rob stayed in couple therapy was perhaps that very early on he could see that Elizabeth was starting to talk about where she was in their relationship. He implied that he wanted to monitor the situation so that he could leave before she did; that was his way of protecting himself from further hurt. Elizabeth spoke about how Rob's service in Vietnam had become a "third person" in their relationship. This was not the way Rob saw it. He felt that his PTSD was a condition or psychiatric disorder that needed to be given more space in the relationship. He could recount terrible things that had happened to him in Vietnam, and most of these stories of terror and horror were related to his witnessing the torture of enemy soldiers and even civilians. As an involuntary witness, he had felt powerless to intervene, and it was this sense of powerlessness that also seemed to permeate his anger with his wife, Elizabeth, over her seeming inability to discipline her children and to unequivocally select him as her top priority. The literature on war zone traumas notes that witnessing or participating in abusive violence or torture appears to create multidimensional traumas that "pose the most complex and difficult therapeutic challenges" (Fontana et al., 1992, p. 754).

These were the obvious issues to work on in the early stabilization phase of the couple therapy. The therapist tried, initially, to help the couple to view the role of the traumatic war service from a shared perspective and to build a more solid rapport between Rob and Elizabeth. It also seemed vital to construct a sense of confidence in the process of couple therapy. Rob made it clear that because the therapist was not a veteran and "If you haven't been there, you can't know," he was only very reluctantly agreeing to attend the couple therapy sessions.

Rob seemed intent on holding Elizabeth at bay and clearly displayed an avoidant and fearful attachment style. Elizabeth, on the other hand, was very anxiously attached to Rob, and she worried constantly about how she would appear in his eyes. The fact that her teenage children were also in the process of separating from her exacerbated her sense of imminent loss and her fear of losing the attachment to Rob. The negative cycle of interaction that could be clearly identified in the early stages of the therapy was Elizabeth's relentless pursuit of signs of emotional connection with Rob (with occasional moments of giving up and turning away) and Rob's emotional withdrawal and withholding of caring gestures and intimate exchanges unless Elizabeth constantly proved her unswerving commitment and loyalty.

Among the sacrifices that Elizabeth imagined she had to make in order to attract Rob's attention, her involvement with her children was high on the list. She understood that Rob often chose to drown his sorrows in alcohol rather than risk connecting with her. She had already seen that Rob could emotionally disconnect himself from his own children, who were independent adults before he came into her life. By the time the couple came for therapy, her eldest child had left home and was attending a university, but Elizabeth also had a teenage son named Mike, who was still at home and appeared to be very demanding of his mother's attention.

STAGE 1. STABILIZATION: PROCESS STEPS AND KEY EVENTS

In the early stage of the couple therapy there seemed to be several areas of concern. First, from Rob's perspective, there appeared to be three main issues: the level of trust Rob could have in Elizabeth if she did not abandon her overt and covert mothering of Mike; his sense of safety about his place in this marriage and in this family, which was a step-family for him, if there was so little recognition of his "sick vet" role; and his alcohol abuse, of which he stoutly maintained he was in complete control. Furthermore, he asserted that he drank only to recapture the sense of camaraderie he had cherished in Vietnam and had not been able to experience since, even with Elizabeth. Early in the sessions he talked about his own sense of being "the villain" in the family. He also stated he could not tolerate seeing or listening to his wife's tearful pleas to be taken into consideration in the relationship.

From Elizabeth's perspective, the issues were radically different. First, she felt that the true enemy in the marriage was the Vietnam War and its continuing hold on Rob. She would attend reunions of the veterans with Rob, but always had a queasy feeling that he was more comfortable with "these drunks," who told maudlin war stories, than he was with her. Rob commented that he did not, in fact, feel close to his veteran buddies, but at least he knew "how to be with them." He added, "It's like I'm in a familiar role, so I feel comfortable—well, more comfortable anyway." In addition, Elizabeth felt personally threatened by Rob's easily aroused anger and hypervigilance, and both of these emotions were most evident when he was around other veterans. Elizabeth's distress was best exemplified by her discomfort with the guns under the marital bed. Second, she remained a captive to her son's rebellious behavior as he continued to "up the ante," in terms of their attachment, and to probe her sense of commitment to him. Third, she thought herself justified in withdrawing into her religious preoccupations when she felt abandoned by Rob, especially when he was drinking and was unavailable to her emotionally or physically.

In these early stages of therapy, the therapist believed it was vital to work on decreasing Rob's reliance on his veteran buddies and to help him focus on other avenues in his life where he could increase his sense of personal mastery and his connection with his partner. The psychiatrist whom Rob continued to see for individual therapy supported this approach. The therapist consulted only once with this psychiatrist at the beginning of therapy, but Rob kept the therapist abreast of what was going on in his individual therapy sessions. That work seemed to center on Rob's going back to school and looking for a job in the social services area, and during the course of therapy Rob did complete his social sciences degree.

As the sessions continued and Rob became more engaged with his partner, he began to spend less time drinking with his veteran buddies. He began to put less emphasis on his role as a war veteran, and this gave Elizabeth a sense of hope as she encouraged Rob to become more involved in other friendships and in her church. Rob started to develop an awareness of how little time he actually spent with Elizabeth and to initiate more activities with her. Although Elizabeth welcomed his refocusing, she remained wary of relying on Rob's attention, because she could not let herself trust in its longevity or its safety. She also worried about her obligations toward her teenage son, who was also interested in spending "alone time" with her.

As the couple talked about the cycle of pursuit, on Elizabeth's part, followed by angry testing and withdrawal by Rob, Rob's potentially violent expressions of anger arose as another issue that had to be dealt with. Elizabeth admitted that she always felt she was "walking on eggshells" around Rob. She was terrified of stirring up his rage with her about some oversight or unintended innuendo. In the early sessions, Elizabeth was often emotional and despondent about her own sense of failing to stand up to Rob and her fear of his reprisal. In the safety of the sessions, she was able to voice a strong sense of not wanting to become the kind of "ghost" that she felt her mother-in-law had become, because she too lived in fear of the ire of her World War II veteran husband.

This admission by Elizabeth truly stunned Rob. He was surprised that she thought he was trying to model himself on his father, whom he secretly feared and did not wish to emulate. Rob told Elizabeth that he thought he would win approval from his tough veteran father if he enlisted for war, and the only war going on at that time was the Vietnam War—not even a war with which Canada was involved. Instead, his father was derisive, calling the Vietnam War a "dirty little jungle *police action*" and describing his son's experience as a teenage adventure in a war that was not a "real" war. Rob wept openly when he talked of his inability to win his father's respect even though he had been severely injured in war and had recovered from his injuries determined to return for a second tour of duty. Rob acknowledged that he was like his father in that he exerted power in his relationship with Elizabeth by insisting that she check all of her decision-making processes with him. Addressing Rob, Elizabeth said that all of her emotions, whether joy, anger, or fear, "have to be filtered through you." Rob would let her know whether a particular feeling was suitable for her to have and to express—or not. She remembered thinking for years that this was obviously the way to keep Rob calm, and with two young children in the house it was important to her that he remain calm. When he became upset with her, and this happened in the sessions, he would talk about writing off the marriage and how he would have to have a contingency plan in place (like a battle plan) for when she would leave him or when he would leave her.

Elizabeth became increasingly able to talk about how she placated and appeased Rob and how even then her own needs often went unheard or misunderstood. Nor did she get the respect she wanted in the relationship. She was able to put Rob's Vietnam experience in a different perspective when she understood that he had been out to show his father that he could be a fearsome warrior and so gain his respect. Her view of the enemy in the relationship shifted from being the war to being Rob's emotionally abusive father and his impact on Rob. She was able to tell Rob how she wanted his respect and a sense of safety and affirmation, just as he longed for these things from his father, and that she did not want to live in fear of Rob's disapproval and threats to leave. Rob began, with the therapist's help, to be able to take in and reflect on her comments.

In turn, Rob disclosed his underlying fears about connecting and depending on someone—anyone. This was just not a safe thing for him to do. So he admitted that he focused on controlling his partner and protecting himself by numbing and withdrawal when emotions got too high. He first learned the danger of depending on an attachment figure when, as a child, he was strapped by his all-powerful father. His need for control and distrust of others was then confirmed in Vietnam, where, he said, "Even your so-called buddies behaved in a barbaric or 'crazy' way that risked your life—the lives of everyone. Enemies were everywhere." Upon his return from Vietnam, he had worked as an inner-city police officer, which further confirmed his sense that people were dangerous. His first wife had also rejected him when he returned from Vietnam, as an "untouchable" killer from a barbaric foreign war. He started to confide that when Elizabeth tried to tell him about her needs, he became very "shaky" because, to him, it meant that he was failing and making a "mess of this attachment too."

The couple now reached the point where their negative cycles of interaction were less dominant in the relationship and both were beginning to move to a new stage where they could talk more directly about their attachment needs and fears. Elizabeth was becoming more assertive, and Rob's sharing about his relationship with his father, and his sense of failure in the relationship with Elizabeth, seemed to open a door to a new level of emotional engagement for him. His sharing of his fears and the need for control that cued his withdrawal from Elizabeth seemed to represent a turning point in therapy.

The couple were now ready to enter Stage 2 of therapy, at which couples begin to rebuild their relational capacities, as described by McCann and Pearlman (1990). From the perspective of emotionally focused couple therapy (EFT), the process of therapy now began to move into reshaping both partners' interactional positions to facilitate more secure bonding. Both Elizabeth and Rob were now able to tolerate and voice feelings they had previously avoided for fear of increasing their alienation from each other. They were able to share that the "aloneness" they often felt was frightening for each of them. It confirmed Rob's sense of unworthiness and all of Elizabeth's insecurities and fears of abandonment and rejection. The following is an excerpt from a session after Rob's sharing of his experience of his relationship with his father and how it had affected his ability to relate to others.

ELIZABETH: If you dislike your father so much, then why do we visit there? I have never liked going there, you know.

ROB: I keep trying to get him to notice me. I want some praise for the person I have become. He has to see it. (*Tears.*)

ELIZABETH: But what if he never does? Does that mean we keep trying, even if that takes time from us as a family?

ROB: What family? (*Puts his hands over his eyes.*) You never make me feel that I belong with you and Mike. I'm always in trouble somehow with the two of you.

THERAPIST: What is it like for you to feel that you don't belong in this family? That you are not making it with Elizabeth either? That must be very hard.

ROB: (*very quiet voice*) I know what Elizabeth will say, but I still don't feel like a flesh and blood person in this family.

THERAPIST: You mean you feel like a ghost in this family? You're never sure you belong. (*Rob nods.*) Elizabeth, isn't that the way you feel when you see how intimidated Rob's mother is by her husband? You see her as a ghost, and you feel like one too as you dance around Rob's anger?

ELIZABETH: Exactly! But I had no idea that Rob felt that way too and that I could have that effect on him.

ROB: Look, this isn't about what is your fault! I just want to feel real in this marriage, as who I am—not just some crazy veteran you're taking pity on and bringing in out of the rain like a stray cat!

THERAPIST: That's your fear, Rob, that Elizabeth just pities you—tolerates you? You can't really believe that she wants and needs you? (*Rob nods and tears.*)

ELIZABETH: Wait a minute. How come this is about you again? What about when I reach for you and you don't feel like flesh and blood to me? You withdraw. You evaporate into thin air.

ROB: (*after a long pause*) Okay, how about this. I'll try to be there for you. I won't withdraw if you try to include me more. I'm not ducking you, really. I'm just doing *my* dance around the ways you can hurt me.

THERAPIST: You are telling Elizabeth that you get afraid that you're not making it with her—that she can't really love a "crazy veteran" and so you put a wall round you? (*Rob nods.*)

ELIZABETH: All I really want is an invitation to the dance—to know I really matter. I don't like being part of the scenery while you play the hero.

ROB: There were no heroes in Vietnam. The place was too full of treachery.

ELIZABETH: Well, I am here, and (*with great emphasis*) I am here now, and I am not trying to betray you.

ROB: (*Sighs and looks down.*) I know . . . I know . . . I know . . .

THERAPIST: It's hard to feel safe isn't it? It feels too fragile for you to trust.

ROB: It's hard even to feel. I've kept my feelings under a flak jacket too long. I can only let out a little at a time. I don't know what it feels like to feel safe. (*Elizabeth reaches out and puts her hand on his arm.*)

STAGE 2. RESTRUCTURING THE BOND

After the discussion involving issues of safety and self-esteem, it felt natural to move on to the development and tolerance of the full spectrum of the relational feelings and cycles of interaction that could foster secure emotional engagement and a positive sense of self for both partners. The goal was for Elizabeth to be able to assert her needs in a way that empowered her and helped Rob to respond to her, and for Rob to risk engagement without his "flak jacket" and his anger at hand.

Earlier, we had tackled two primary issues in their relationship: One was his authoritarian stance with his step-son, and the other was the role that the symptoms of PTSD played in their relationship. With regard to Mike, Rob was willing to acknowledge that Elizabeth had very protective feelings both toward him and toward her son. Rob further admitted that he did not like to see Elizabeth sad, and when her son was rebellious and rude and made her sad, then Rob became very angry with him. As we delved into these feelings, other feelings of insecurity emerged for Rob.

At these times, Rob worried that Elizabeth would leave him. He clearly saw his role as being the family provider and protector, and that gave him a solid, secure place to stand in this step-family. Mike represented a threat to that place to stand. If Rob could not protect Elizabeth and control his step-son's rebellious behavior, then, by his own criteria, he had failed. He then expected Elizabeth to see him as a pathetic failure and abandon him. He also pointed out to her that she would inevitably end up taking Mike's side and, effectively, leave Rob to "twist in the wind." When Elizabeth tried to talk more about this, she shared that when she became intimidated by his expressions of anger, she did "deaden" her feelings for him. This admission immediately caused Rob to be very angry, and he resorted again to talking about his contingency plans to protect himself should the relationship fail. However, when supported by the therapist, he was able to listen to Elizabeth and recognize echoes of his own feelings of engulfing sadness, emotional numbness, and pervasive sense of dread. He began to talk more about his fears of failing her and losing her.

Elizabeth tried very hard to communicate to Rob that she needed him to understand that when she felt threatened by his anger, she then moved to protect her son from this anger. But she did understand his dilemma and did want his support with Mike. She was able to be clear, with the therapist's help, that she did not see Rob as a "crazed Nam vet," that, in fact, she got scared of her own anger with her son. Rob then became very agitated and brought up what seemed like a new topic. He began to talk of how Elizabeth had taken their sick old dog to be put down. When asked by the therapist to connect the threads here, he stated that it was obvious and no wonder he got "scared." The following dialogue then evolved, which demonstrates Rob's beginning to risk being more vulnerable and open to a more engaged Elizabeth:

THERAPIST: (*very softly*) What are you scared of?

ROB: I guess, well, if it was so easy for her to kill the dog, what would she do to me if she knew . . . (*Puts his face in his hands.*)

THERAPIST: (*softly again*) Knew what?

ROB: (*very quietly*) That I don't love Mike the way she wants me to (*long silence*). He's trouble. I know it. He is going to hurt her badly because he is irresponsible. He could never have survived in Nam. He would have been picked off early. I get so angry that he is so careless and casual about stuff.

ELIZABETH: Rob, I am not leaving, and I know how hard Mike can be. But I'm afraid to get angry with Mike in front of you. You always outdo me in that department, and then what will happen to Mike?

THERAPIST: If you can't protect Mike from himself and stop him from hurting Elizabeth, then you will disappoint her and . . .

ROB: I will lose her. It always boils down to that, doesn't it? (*Therapist nods.*) So I numb out or threaten. And I get obsessed with "survival," I guess. If Mike doesn't survive, she'll never forgive me.

Elizabeth then began to expand on her understanding of Rob's anger and its complex etiology and expression, which were so intimately connected to his feelings about safety. Rob was also able to respond to Elizabeth's concern about his anger and hear how she would like to be supported in regard to her son. Part of this exchange involved Rob's grappling with his own black-and-white view of the world, which had been initiated at home and confirmed in war. He had developed a self-styled profound and unarguable sense of right and wrong. In part, such angry insistence on doing what is right is a reflection of what Jonathan Shay (1994) refers to as the reaction of *menis* (indignant wrath) to any act construed as a violation of *themis*, or that which is right. He suggests that this response is particularly found in combat veterans. Elizabeth saw Rob's stance as a demand for justice and retribution. She spoke about how she became anxious and tried to calm and placate Rob when he took a rigid moral stance, but, feeling emotionally shunned by him, would finally give up and withdraw into activities for a while.

Elizabeth's anxious and Rob's fearful-avoidant attachment styles, and the part his displays of anger played in the maintenance of these styles, became apparent in a dramatic incident that happened midway through therapy. It was an example of how, in this work of promoting safe emotional engagement with couples who have a history of traumatic experiences and emotionally corroded attachment bonds, the therapist is often in the position of snatching little nuggets of victory from the jaws of defeat. After a great session in which Rob had begun to confront the impact of his anger on the relationship, Rob and Mike had gotten into an argument at home. Rob had taken an impulsive swipe at Mike and just missed hitting him on the jaw.

ROB: (*pushing out his jaw*) If the kid is going to be that rude, then he is going to get a fat lip.

ELIZABETH: (*to therapist*) Mike really provoked Rob. Well, I too have felt like slapping Mike for his insolence. The worst happened, and we all survived. Amazing!

ROB: What are you talking about? I nearly hit the kid! I am a really bad father. I did what I vowed I would never do. I reminded myself of my father. Oh God . . . (*Puts his head in his hands.*)

THERAPIST: Do you remember what you felt just before you took that swing at Mike?

ROB: Yeah . . . I was thinking, here we go again. . . . It's like Nam. I felt so powerless, like such a failure when I could not get the torture to stop. This stuff . . . it's all my dark side . . . it's bad stuff, and usually I can keep it away from my life now.

ELIZABETH: (*sighs; then in a soft voice*) Are we never to be done with it, what happened to you in Vietnam and your anger? Do we have to keep paying for it over and over again?

THERAPIST: (*to Elizabeth*) Maybe this isn't so much about anger. Maybe this is more about loss of innocence and an overwhelming sense of failure and powerlessness?

ELIZABETH: We all fail in life. It's just that some of us do it in a jungle and some of us do it as mothers . . . or wives. (*Begins to cry.*)

ROB: (*in a patient and soothing voice*) I'm sorry that the dark side of me comes out, and I can understand that it makes you want to cry. It makes me cry too for that gung-ho kid that went to Vietnam and came back old and bitter. (*Tears.*)

ELIZABETH: (*with a soft voice*) Are you crying for me or with me?

ROB: I'm crying for me, for you too, but . . . finally, for me . . .

Rob then asked for her comfort and reassurance, and Elizabeth comforted him.

During and after this session, both partners faced the fire of Rob's rage and torment with his own feelings of helplessness, and they both began to feel safe in expressing their feelings about Mike and other stressors in their lives without fear of emotional or attachment reprisal. They also began to feel more comfortable with the idea of backing each other up when Mike continued to pull typical teenager stunts.

In terms of Rob managing his PTSD in the relationship, the second issue that came up was Rob's drinking. Rob was working very hard during this time to eliminate his drinking. This was difficult for him, but he wanted to convince himself that he had control over alcohol. Elizabeth was able to tell him that it was not his drinking (which was not always excessive) she had the problem with, but his rage and "black-and-white" attitude when he did, as he put it, "slip up with the drinking." The couple started to become more mutually accepting and philosophical about the ups and downs of living and loving together, including the "sparks" of PTSD and the occasional drinking lapses. The couple began to construct a "healing theory" (Figley, 1989), that framed their relationship as bigger than Rob's trauma and the challenges of their everyday life. Rob began to be able to talk to Elizabeth about his understanding that the essence of trauma is the overwhelming sense of being absolutely helpless, and that if this feeling was sparked, he responded with "desperate" measures. We talked about his experience when he rolled over a land mine in a jeep and his sense of helplessness when he was pinned under the jeep and an enemy patrol came by. There was nothing he could do but pretend to be dead. From this discussion we got into a conversation about how traumatic events can render you helpless and really blow a big hole in your life. Rob was able to identify times when relationship cues sparked off his "helplessness" and sense of imminent loss, and times when he really needed Elizabeth's comfort and support. He began to talk about how Elizabeth's touch could stop his "free fall into despair and the helplessness that comes from being so alone."

A final issue in this stage of therapy arose when Rob announced that he had decided that they should move to a remote country area where he had been offered a job and where life was "safer" and he could put a "fence around my land." Elizabeth became very upset in the session and stated that she had not been consulted and did not want to go. The following dialogue evolved:

ROB: (to Elizabeth) You're stammering, and it's really annoying that you can't express yourself in complete sentences.

THERAPIST: Rob, do you have any sense of how loud and angry you sound right now?

ROB: Angry? I'm not angry now. You want to see me angry? I can be so angry I can tear your office apart.

THERAPIST: Yes, well, I really don't want you to do that, but I think you need to know that I'm feeling very uncomfortable because you are sounding so angry. I really don't know what is going to happen next. You talk like you have nothing to lose here.

ROB: (*Becomes calmer and seems to be musing as he speaks.*) Nothing to lose; nothing to lose. She's sitting there crying, and you're telling me I have nothing to lose. She is my life. Nothing is any good without her. I want to go and be at peace with her in the country where we can't be disturbed or hurt.

ELIZABETH: If you only weren't still so angry sometimes. I refuse to keep walking on eggshells around you. I feel so tired.

ROB: You're tired. How do you think I feel? Every time I try to talk to you, it's as if I have to go through this screen of your tears. I thought you were going to be different. (*Turns to the therapist.*) When I met her, she lived in this cottage in the woods and she seemed so at ease there in the woods. It felt so safe to get close to her back then. She seemed so calm.

THERAPIST: Do you ever get that feeling now about her calmness?

ROB: Yes, I sometimes get it when I look across the table at her on Christmas Day.

THERAPIST: So that is a really good feeling for you?

ROB: All the goodness in my life is connected to her. She used to be able to let my anger just wash over her.

THERAPIST: I see. So you want Elizabeth to just duck when you are angry and let the anger wash over her, and then she can emerge as a calm, supportive listener to you. Is that what you want? (*Rob nods but smiles. He knows this request is unreasonable.*)

THERAPIST: Elizabeth, how do you feel about that?

ELIZABETH: It just makes me feel really, really tired. I could do that sometimes, but what do I do when his anger is washing over me and feels like it's just going to keep coming and it's drowning me? That's scary.

ROB: (*quietly*) Well, I guess that means I'm just a screwup and I'm not going to be able to do anything about it. I'm just bad, and eventually I'm out of this relationship too.

ELIZABETH: No, I want you to slow down here. No, that's not what I want and you know that now, and I don't believe it's what you want either. And you have been able to step aside and limit the anger recently.

THERAPIST: You are telling him you need him to do that? (*Elizabeth nods emphatically.*) What do you think, Rob? Do you believe Elizabeth is going to hang in with you? (*Rob and Elizabeth exchange a long glance and smile at each other.*) Can you tell her how important she is to you?

ROB: She's my ears. She has always been able to hear scary noises in the house, because I lost some of my hearing in Vietnam. She lets me know if I need to get upset about things. She's my early warning device.

THERAPIST: You really count on her. (*Rob nods.*) She is your safety. But what about when Elizabeth gets upset with you and she scares you? Can she tell you now that she is scared?

ROB: I would never really hurt her. I don't want her to be frightened, especially not of me, but she seems to go off somewhere.

THERAPIST: Elizabeth, do you know what Rob is talking about when he says you go off somewhere?

ELIZABETH: Well, I guess I try so hard to reach him, or make contact or placate him. But if I can't, well, then I kind of, maybe I kind of blank out. I pretend I'm not there. I go into myself and ask myself questions, and I give myself answers, and that's how I calm myself. It's so I can stay with him really, stay and wait till he calms down.

ROB: But when you are off in your own little world, I feel so completely alone. I don't have anyone to let me know whether or not the situation is really dangerous or not.

THERAPIST: So you get scared sometimes by Elizabeth, by how upset she gets, and then you feel like you've failed, or is it her distance that really scares you?

ROB: Both, yes. But especially her distance. Then I feel really, really . . .

THERAPIST: Helpless?

ROB: Right. I feel like I drive her away—don't want to do that.

THERAPIST: Can you tell her that, Rob?

ROB: (*Turns to Elizabeth.*) I don't want to drive you away (*long pause*). Look, this is not that hard to get. I want to be with you in a safe place, it doesn't have to be the country, and I want to take care of you. I need you to be my ears—my safety. You know you already have all my heart. (*Leans forward and reaches out for Elizabeth; she responds. They hug.*)

STAGE 3. CONSOLIDATION AND INTEGRATION

The couple began to be able to create predictable sequences of comfort and closeness and to quickly step out of negative cycles of interaction when they did occur. They were able to construct a clear narrative of their relationship history and how they had changed this relationship in therapy. They could now reflect on and joke about their present dance with all its pitfalls. They spoke of the teeter-totter of their relationship and how ups and downs were inevitable, but now less threatening for their relationship. Rob began to talk about how, if you are going to live around the edges of the black hole of trauma, you need to expand your safe territory as much as you can and to stop yourself from falling back into the hole. The best way to do that, he said, is to build a picket fence around the hole. The pickets Rob could use to build that fence were safe, secure attachment figures, like Elizabeth, and his other interests in life that gave him the feeling of mastery and assurance. He now felt that he was not helpless to reconstitute his life and his sense of who he was. For Rob, as he formulated it, Elizabeth was the essential picket to protect him from that long free fall into the black hole of despair and loneliness that had opened in his childhood and grew deeper and darker in Vietnam. The work he was doing with a drop-in center for young people definitely gave him a sense of efficacy, because he felt useful and fulfilled working with these disenfranchised youngsters, who expressed their appreciation to him for his care and concern.

Elizabeth talked about how she often felt that she failed in her role as "Rob's picket." Even though she would try every way she could think of to make him feel safe, to help him to trust her, she could not do it. Then the hole seemed to be getting bigger and bigger, and they were both in it. She talked about what she could or was willing to do and what she could not do. She had decided that she would have to trust Rob to deal with his own issues, including the allure of drinking. She was also able to reiterate that she could not always help him feel safe and was *not* willing to be tested continually in this regard. However, she also felt much stronger in being able to say what she needed, and this helped her to stay closer to Rob and support him. She saw herself becoming a stronger person in that she could let Rob know that she would not accept his ever returning to heavy drinking or bouts of uncontrolled anger. She now expected him to be able to talk about his fears and needs, so that those angry outbursts, if they occurred at all, were brief and less intense. She said that she saw that he now seemed able to do this. However, Elizabeth then also informed Rob that she now expected him to take care of his alcohol addiction once and for all by getting professional help immediately. He agreed.

The couple were able to identify "hot spots" in their relationship that they needed to contain and ways to comfort and reassure each other when either became anxious. With the therapist's help, they also talked more about Rob's sense that he lived on borrowed time and how this influenced the way he planned for the future. He had had this sense ever since he survived the accident in Vietnam. Elizabeth had never paid much attention to this sense of doom or to Rob's feeling that he was not entitled to have good things in life. Part of him believed that if he tried to have something good in his life, it would inevitably be snatched away from him. He was always watching and waiting for loss and disaster, so it was hard for him to share in Elizabeth's plans for the future. In these sessions, the couple were demonstrably affectionate with each other and both told of incidents that they saw as evidence of the new patterns in their relationship. Elizabeth recounted an incident when she had approached Rob during the week to say that she needed to talk about something that was bothering her and he had listened carefully. They then talked about Elizabeth's sense that she was becoming more comfortable in the relationship and was most often able to offer Rob the support he needed. Likewise, Rob was more responsive to Elizabeth's needs and had taken care of her after a recent minor operation. He also acknowledged that now he did not need to get into a panic if she saw something completely differently from the way he viewed it. A difference between them was no longer a cue for imminent loss. These final interactions were viewed as very positive by both partners, as well as representative of the new connection between their "stronger" selves.

The couple continued to talk about how the symptoms of PTSD could, on occasion, interfere with their marriage, but they talked about it with more humor than bitterness. They spoke of how, even in the face of such symptoms, they could still fill each other's lives with compassion, trust, and confidence as they continued to learn how to create safe intimacy in the shadow of the dragon of trauma. There was a place where they could stand together.

Chapter 10

Relationship Traumas: Attachment Injuries in Close Relationships

" 'Never again,' I told myself. He would never do that to me again."

*A*ttachment theorists have pointed out that because of the profound psychological and physiological interdependence involved in attachment bonds, incidents in which one partner responds or fails to respond at times of urgent need seem to disproportionately influence the quality of an attachment relationship (Simpson & Rholes, 1994). Negative attachment-related events, particularly abandonments and betrayals, often cause seemingly irreparable damage to close relationships. Many partners enter therapy not only in general distress, but also with the goal of bringing closure to such events and so restoring lost intimacy and trust. During the therapy process, however, these events, referred to here as attachment injuries, often reemerge still very much alive and intensely emotional and—much like a traumatic flashback—overwhelm the injured partner. When the other partner then fails to respond in a reparative, reassuring manner or when the injured spouse cannot accept such reassurance, the injury is then compounded. As the couple experience failure in their attempts to move beyond such injuries and repair the bond between them, their despair and alienation deepen.

181

So, a partner's withdrawal from his wife while she suffers a miscarriage, as well as his subsequent unwillingness to discuss this incident and address his wife's hurt related to the incident, becomes a recurring focus of the couple's dialogue and blocks the development of new, more positive interactions. This incident then becomes a central, defining event in the couple's relationship and influences how the partners emotionally engage each other.

The couple therapy literature has recently attempted to deal with particular kinds of betrayals or relationship traumas that make repair of a relationship more difficult. There has been much discussion of infidelity, for example, and how to help couples deal with such events (Abrams Spring, 1997). The literature on forgiveness is relevant here (Enright & Fitzgibbons, 2000; Flanigan, 1992; Worthington & DiBlasio, 1990). However, there seems to be little understanding of the specific nature of the kinds of negative events that call for forgiveness, which is often defined as an intrapersonal rather than an interpersonal process. Nor have views of forgiveness been integrated into broader theories of marriage (Coop Gordon, Baucom, & Snyder, 2000). Perhaps because of this lack of a broad theoretical framework, there is little consensus as to the critical elements of forgiveness and how and why particular kinds of negative incidents impact relationships in particular ways.

The concept of attachment injury does not focus so much on the specific content of a painful event, but on the attachment significance of such events. Some incidents involving some form of infidelity may be experienced as attachment injuries, whereas other incidents may not. As mentioned previously, attachment theory has been called a theory of trauma (Atkinson, 1997) in that it emphasizes the extreme emotional adversity of isolation and separation, particularly at times of increased vulnerability. Such isolation, especially at these times, evokes the sense of helplessness that is the essence of the trauma experience. This theoretical framework offers an explanation of why certain events become pivotal in a relationship, as well as an indication of what the key features of such events will be, how they will affect a particular couple's relationship, and how such events can be optimally resolved. Although these events may be considered small-"t" traumas, rather than the life-shaping events to which this term usually refers, they are nevertheless extremely significant. Like the more jarring traumatic events, they overwhelm coping capacities and define the experience, in this case the relationship, as a source of danger rather than a safe haven in times of stress.

This concept of attachment injury emerged from the observation of impasses in the therapy process with couples whose relationship improved but did not recover from distress in emotionally focused couple therapy (EFT). Observations of the process with couples who did not respond optimally to therapy revealed a clear pattern. As the more withdrawn partner became more accessible and the therapist began to encourage the other, more blaming, partner to risk trusting and confiding, an emotionally laden incident, often first described at the beginning of therapy, would become the focus of the session. As the therapist fostered the confiding of attachment vulnerabilities and needs, for example, a partner would balk and hark back to a specific incident of betrayal, whereas the other partner might discount or not even remember the event. This incident sometimes appeared, at first glance, to be relatively insignificant, but it evoked compelling, constricted emotional responses and rigid interaction patterns, such as blame–defend, that blocked further progress. Partners used the language of trauma when describing such injuries. They spoke in life-and-death terms. They spoke of isolation and abandonment. A past violation of trust would be described, and the injured party would take a stance of "never again," refusing to risk becoming vulnerable to the other. The other partner would then become angry or withdraw. Unless the therapist could find ways to help the couple deal with this perceived violation of trust, the couple would then be unable to create the positive cycles and bonding events found in the sessions of more successful couples (Johnson & Greenberg, 1988).

At what point do these injuries usually arise in therapy? Once the relationship has stabilized in therapy and partners are able to use their emotional experiences as guides to their needs and communicate these needs in a way that maximizes the other's responsiveness, the interactional dance begins to change. A withdrawn partner, now able to explore the emotional experiences that evoke his or her withdrawal, becomes more emotionally engaged. The more hostile partner becomes able to express his or her hurts and fears and to take new risks with the other partner. It is at this point, however, as partners are invited to step into a new dance, a dance in which they put themselves in each other's hands, that attachment injuries are particularly likely to come alive with all the intensity of a traumatic flashback.

Couples are sometimes clear, right from the first session, that specific past attachment-related events marked a shift in the bond between them and continue to define the relationship. Injured partners may refer to such events and use them as proof of their partners' inadequacies and failings in the relationship. An argument may then ensue about what occurred and what meaning should be assigned to the event. It appears that these kinds of wounds to the attachment bond cannot be left behind, nor can they be resolved in the negative emotional climate of the first stage of therapy. Indeed, some partners do not even bring up these events until later in therapy. In any case, it is usually not until the therapist begins to encourage partners to share their vulnerabilities and emotionally engage on this level that these events move to front and center. They must then be dealt with, if the couple is to reconfigure their relationship as a secure bond in which each can be vulnerable and open about his or her needs for comfort and care. If such events cannot be resolved, trust remains tentative, positive bonding cycles are more circumscribed, and relapse into relationship distress is a greater possibility.

ATTACHMENT INJURIES AS RELATIONSHIP TRAUMAS

An attachment injury is a specific type of betrayal experienced in couple relationships, characterized as an abandonment or a violation of trust (Johnson & Whiffen, 1999). It is not a general trust issue. It concerns a specific incident in which one partner is inaccessible and unresponsive in the face of the other partner's urgent need for the kind of support and caring expected of attachment figures. *It is a potential prototypical bonding scenario that turns into the nightmare of finding oneself alone when one is most helpless and most desperate.* The injurious incident is then continually used as a touchstone as to the dependability of the other partner. Such events, if unresolved, not only damage the nature of the attachment bond between the couple, they prevent the repair of this bond.

The actual incident that precipitates an attachment injury is not necessarily the primary causal factor in a couple's marital distress. Some partners may have endured insecure or frayed attachment bonds over a period of years and for a number of reasons. One incident in particular may then exacerbate this distress and act as a symbolic marker of insecure attachment for the injured partner. Another couple may have had a relatively secure bond up to the time when this kind of incident occurs. The injury then marks the beginning of their relational distress, in that it shatters the assumptions of a bonding relationship and plunges the injured individual into emotional isolation.

Different forms of attachment injuries experienced by couples must be considered. Some may appear trivial or exaggerated to an outsider, or they may be more obvious betrayals of trust, such as infidelity. Feelings of abandonment and betrayal may emerge at any time when one partner fails to respond to the other at moments when attachment needs are particularly salient. These moments most often occur during times of transition, loss, physical danger, and existential uncertainty. Classic examples of such times are the birth of a child, times of physical illness (for example, after a cancer diagnosis), times of disorienting life transitions (such as retirement or immigration), and times of loss (miscarriage or the death of a child).

Moreover, what may be a manageable hurt for one couple may be a momentous interpersonal cataclysm for another. A man who has recently lost his job and then has been told that he is infertile and unable to father a child, and whose wife, in an argument, tells him that she will find a man who is more potent, flushes red and wrings his hands when he speaks of his wife's pronouncement. He also brings up this event and becomes either extremely hostile or "terrorized" and disoriented when he is encouraged in any way to confide in his wife. Another man, at another time, with another individual history or with a different kind of relationship dance with a different partner, may have been less traumatized or better able to deal with his hurt in a more flexible way that left the relationship relatively unharmed. This incident, however, dramatically altered the way the reality of this infertile couple's relationship was defined, in the same way that trauma alters the world of individual victims.

Much depends on how the injured partner interprets the event in question and how his or her spouse responds to the injured party's expressions of hurt. When the spouse discounts, denies, or dismisses the injury, it prevents the processing of the event in the relationship and compounds the injury. The unresolved event may be the topic of constant bickering, or it may lay dormant and unexpressed for a period of time. However, it eventually reemerges with a vengeance, especially when a subsequent incident evokes an emotional response related to the initial injury.

A couple were referred to therapy because the husband's retirement had precipitated a clinical depression and marital distress. When the couple came in, however, the main problem seemed to be the wife's angry unwillingness to engage in activities with her husband. As he was encouraged by the therapist to ask his wife for hugs and physical affection, his wife exploded. She then explained, with quiet intensity, that she did not intend to respond to him. She asked whether he remembered that exactly 16 years ago, on a particular winter afternoon, he had returned from work to find her in the kitchen, ill and depressed and trying to care for three very small children? Did he recall that she had desperately begged him to hold her for a moment, or that he had instead gone off to make a series of long phone calls? She had then collapsed and, in her despair, promised herself never to ask him for comfort again. She had kept this promise and had immersed herself in bringing up her children. He did not recall this incident, and she had never discussed it with him. As she described the incident, however, she flushed, wrung her hands, and wept as if it had occurred just yesterday.

Attachment injuries can be clearly distinguished from the ordinary highs and lows of an ongoing relationship. It seems most useful to view them as relationship traumas. *Trauma* is a Latin word meaning "wound" or "injury," and "to injure" comes from the Latin word *injuria*, meaning "to wrong" (Walser & Hayes, 1998). Not all painful events are traumatic or evoke a sense of being wronged or betrayed. Traumatic experience shatters assumptions, changes the way we see ourselves and others, and induces a sense of existential vulnerability.

Betrayals such as attachment injuries call into question a person's basic beliefs about relationships, the other, and the self. As partners commit to an intimate relationship, they have an internal model of what the relationship will look like and how they expect to be treated. Couples typically expect their partners to be attentive, responsive, and supportive, especially in times of crisis. More specific expectations (i.e., time spent together, socializing, division of domestic labor, etc.) evolve from the everyday relationship experiences. Under normal circumstances the violation of expectations does not necessarily harm the essential nature of the attachment bond; however, when a person is most vulnerable and comfort is essential, such violations can rupture the bond significantly.

When a partner cries out for help in extreme need and there is no response, the sense of basic trust in the other is shattered. The most basic assumption of attachment relationships, that my partner will be there for me when needed, is suddenly destroyed. The shattering of this basic assumption is, in and of itself, disorienting and is part of the sense of helplessness that is perhaps the most salient feature of traumatic experience. Such a violation may also constitute a serious threat to assumptions about the self. A client once stated, "I was just not that important to him. I wasn't precious. My hurt didn't matter." When one partner fails to respond to another's basic dependency needs, this threatens not only the injured partner's sense of security in the world but also his or her sense of self-worth. This hurt is compounded when the injuring partner then refuses to acknowledge or deal with the injured person's pain.

Attachment theory states that when people are without physical or emotional support, they are at their most vulnerable and have most difficulty regulating their emotions. Disturbances of affect are central to all descriptions of traumatic stress and its sequelae. In therapy, couples often talk about these injurious events with overwhelming emotion, and most often speak in terms of life and death (e.g., "I was so sick I could have died," "You watched me drown," "You didn't care that I crashed and burned after that argument"). Following traumatic abandonment, an injured partner's involvement in the relationship often becomes organized around eliciting emotional responsiveness, or defending against the lack of this responsiveness from the other partner. Moreover, the injured partner may exhibit the classic symptoms characteristic of PTSD, such as re-experiencing, numbness, and hypervigilance.

Re-experiencing traumatic events emanates from the "indelible imprint" of the traumatic moment (Herman, 1992, p. 35). Memories and emotions connected to the event linger and manifest themselves in the form of dreams, flashbacks, and intrusive memories in relationship traumas, as in individual traumas. Much energy may be spent in ruminating about every minute detail of the event and the reasons that it occurred. Offending partners sometimes apologize for their transgressions, but injured partners cannot let the matter go. These events are pivotal moments in the ongoing definition of the relationship that constantly come up and color present realities.

Avoidance and numbing, the natural self-protective responses to a barrage of intrusive trauma symptoms, can be very costly for a relationship. Numbing prevents emotional engagement with the partner and so interferes with resolution of the attachment injury. An alternating sequence of numbing, intrusive images, and hyperarousal is a response to the paralyzing attachment paradox perceived by the injured party. As attachment theorists (Main & Hesse, 1990) have pointed out, situations in which the primary attachment figure is at once a source of and a solution to pain and fear are inherently difficult to tolerate and result in a fundamental disorganization of the attachment system. The injured party tends to swing between hypo- and hyperarousal, first accusing and clinging, then numbing and withdrawing. This pattern then becomes chaotic and aversive to both partners. Even when the injured spouse can elicit comfort from the other, he or she does not trust it. The open confiding that allows us to give meaning and structure to difficult experiences (Pennebaker, 1985) is also almost impossible. *In short, the couple's ways of coping with the attachment injury become aversive in themselves and perpetuate the alienation between them.* Physiological hyperarousal, another cardinal symptom of PTSD, reflects the persistent expectation of impending danger. Relatively subtle echoes of the relationship trauma tends to evoke extreme fight, flight, and freeze responses. Exaggerated sensitivities and hypervigilance for further signs of betrayal then become the norm. Normally positive interactions become tentative and colored by doubts. The couple are then caught in a drama in which the injured spouse sets tests and the offending spouse is always found wanting. The following sections consider a specific example of an attachment injury and how it appears in couple therapy.

AN ATTACHMENT INJURY STORY:
THE CASE OF LOU AND JOHN

John, a successful lawyer, and Lou, a professional artist, had been married for 14 years. They had no children and described relationship interactions characterized by withdraw–withdraw. Until about 2 years ago, Lou had pursued John for closeness, while he remained "cold" and reserved. Since Lou had "shut down," however, they had become, in Lou's words, "just distant friends—we go through the motions is all. Our relationship is a no-man's-land." John described himself as simply "hunkering down" and avoiding confrontation. He agreed that he had become so good at "chilling out" that he no longer knew how he felt. At the end of the first session, Lou began to describe their past experience of couple therapy and a particularly "catastrophic" session when "something had snapped" and she had "switched off," so that she now took very few risks with John and allowed distancing to take over the relationship. In an individual session with Lou, it became clear that the session in question had involved an attachment injury for Lou. She became very shaky and distressed as she described how John and the male therapist had agreed in this session that she was "too needy" and had to accommodate to John's relational style. She described herself as feeling "betrayed and violated" and as being depressed and suicidal for days after that session. She had then ended the therapy sessions and with-drawn from her husband. She also confided that to return to couple therapy was a huge step for her and that she was watching me to see if I was, in fact, about to do something similar and so betray her.

This incident formed the backdrop to the whole therapy process, emerging occasionally onto center stage. However, once John had be-come re-engaged (or, in his words, "less detached"), and was able to reach for Lou and risk closeness with her consistently, the echoes of this incident became more pervasive and insidious. When John tried to initi-ate closeness, Lou would close her mouth in a tight line and speak of being "bored." She made remarks like, "You carry the relationship. I think I am dropping it." When we explored these responses, she was able to speak of her anger and her unwillingness to expose herself again to the kind of hurt she had felt in the session referred to earlier. As we began to address this issue, the following dialogue evolved:

JOHN: It's because you are so important to me that I freeze up. I want you to give me a chance.

LOU: If I was so important, you wouldn't have shut me out for all those years. And then, when I was really desperate, right on the edge, you did that, in that session. (*Begins to shake. Holds onto the arm of the chair and sobs.*) It was the final blow. (*Holds her head in her hands and turns away.*) (*in a very soft voice*) Everything changed then.

THERAPIST: You are talking about how wounded you were in the final therapy session last year, is that right, Lou? (*Lou nods.*) That is still so painful for you—it's right here—and it comes up when John reaches for you and asks you to open up, to risk and respond to him? (*Lou nods emphatically.*) Have you ever really told him the impact that session had on you?

LOU: A little. I guess I have. He joined with the therapist—the two of them, they just put me in a box and labeled me. I was just infantile, pathetic. That was the message I got, and he went along with it. It got him off the hook, you see.

THERAPIST: You felt discounted, ganged up on, betrayed? Can you tell him . . . ?

LOU: I felt all of that. (*Turns to John.*) You both talked about me like I was a mental case, a nonperson. After all the struggles we had been through—all the times I had tried to get you to talk. You wiped me out. I have never felt so alone, never. Something just snapped and that night—I didn't tell you—I just felt like everything we had together had been a lie. I just felt so devastated. I found myself thinking of really terrible things—about how it would be a relief just to die, because no one was ever going to be there for me. How could you do that to me—to us? (*She weeps.*) And now—now you want me to smile and try again. I grieved for months after that session, and you kept your distance. I promised I would never give you the chance to hurt me like that again. I don't know what I'm doing here.

THERAPIST: (*softly*) You felt abandoned, labeled—more alone than you ever had in your life. (*Lou nods vigorously.*) This haunts you, and you find it hard to even talk about. (*Lou nods again.*) And you promised yourself never to give anyone the chance to hurt you like that again. So now, when John asks you to risk and open up to him, all this hurt and grief and fear comes up. (*turning to John*) What happens to you when you hear this, John?

JOHN: (*Leans toward Lou*) I feel terrible. I let her down. We had talked about it, but I never heard . . . (*long pause*) I let you down. I guess I felt relieved when he said that you had to mature a bit and accept me as I was. I felt relieved to hear him say it wasn't me and I wasn't so bad after all. I didn't want to look at my problems. So I let it unfold. I never knew—(*tears*). I felt relieved—I heard him say that the marriage would be okay. I focused on that—I didn't see . . .

THERAPIST: (*to Lou, who is staring intently out the window*) Can you hear him, Lou? He heard the therapist say the relationship was all right and he hadn't been such a bad spouse—is that okay, John? (*He nods.*) Lou, what is happening to you right now?

LOU: He was the only person I had ever felt close to. (*Puts her head between her hands and whispers.*) And then he wasn't there. I was so desperate—I wanted to die, to give up on the hope of comfort and caring. I wanted to die. I felt like I was disintegrating, coming apart. (*Looks up at John.*) Do you get that?

JOHN: (*very softly and slowly*) I think so. (*Leans forward.*) I am so sorry. I am so sorry, Lou. I let you down—when you needed me, I let you down. (*Cries.*) I didn't get it. I was so caught up in being relieved that I wasn't so bad, as a husband. I'm sorry. I'm so sorry.

THERAPIST: Can you hear him, Lou?

LOU: Kind of. (*Sits back in her chair.*) But a part of me says, "Don't be taken in—don't let yourself hope."

THERAPIST: There is a spark of hope when you hear John respond to your grief and pain, but you want to protect yourself—yes? Can you imagine that you might be able to let John comfort you? (*Lou shakes her head and looks down.*)

JOHN: (*very quietly*) I can understand that you would want to hold back, after all the years I stayed reserved and then—this. I want you to know (*long pause*), I want you to know how desperate I am for you to try to forgive me—I don't want to lose you. You mean everything to me. I will do—whatever you need me to do—I don't want you to give up on us.

THERAPIST: Can you hear him, Lou? Or is it too scary to let that hope and longing for him come up again?

LOU: Yes, it is—it's very scary. I won't ever feel that way again—I felt like I was dying.

Lou then went on to explore her fear of putting herself "in John's hands" again. He remained engaged and comforted and reassured her. She then gradually began to talk of "trying to find a way back to him." Jim acknowledged many times that she had a right to feel angry and hurt by the events in that past therapy session and by his lack of empathy afterward. They began to be able to comfort each other and express relief that they had nearly, but not quite, lost their relationship. Once this injury was resolved, Lou began to be able to take small steps toward John and ask for her needs to be met. John, with my support, was able to respond, and the couple were able to move into the last stage of therapy and consolidate their strengthened bond.

This particular traumatic incident in Lou and John's relationship was not difficult to understand. However, the presentation of such injuries is not always so clear and straightforward. For example, a couple came to therapy with an extreme attack–defend cycle in which the wife would sarcastically berate the husband for many "crimes," but particularly for his recent friendship with a female colleague who was in trouble. She did not suspect an affair and seemed to be irrationally moralistic and accusatory. I began to have difficulty empathizing with this client's position. The wife focused with obsessive concentration on an incident in which her husband offered to go out in a snowstorm and start his colleague's car for her after a party. The picture became clear only when I remembered the wife's brief allusion to returning home after a minor operation during which, for a moment, she had faced death. She reported that she had begun to share her fears with her spouse but he told her that he was exhausted and just had to go to bed. She had never brought up this topic again. I then suggested that the wife could not bear to see her husband give to his colleague the caring and protective soothing that she herself had longed for after her operation but could not directly ask for. The wife responded with an intense, vivid reentry into the experience of the operation and her isolation upon returning home. This was a turning point in the therapy with this couple, and I went on to help the wife address her vulnerability and her contempt for her own attachment needs. The husband was then able to respond to his wife's hurt and fear. The couple were able to resolve the injury and complete the bonding sequences of mutual comfort and caring.

THE RESOLUTION OF ATTACHMENT INJURIES

How are such relationship traumas resolved? The patterns that my colleagues and I have noted in the process of resolution are as follows:

1. A marker denotes the beginning of the event. As the therapist encourages the injured spouse to begin to risk connecting with the more accessible partner, this spouse begins to describe an incident in which he or she felt abandoned and helpless, experiencing a violation of trust that damaged his or her belief in the relationship as a secure bond. This spouse speaks of the incident in a highly emotional, often disjointed manner. The incident is alive and present, rather than a calm recollection. The partner often either discounts, denies, or minimizes the incident and the injured spouse's pain and moves to a defensive stance.

2. With the therapist's help, the injured spouse stays in touch with the injury and begins to articulate its impact and it attachment significance. New emotions frequently emerge at this point. Anger evolves into clear expressions of hurt, helplessness, fear, and shame. The connection of the injury to present negative cycles in the relationship become clear. For example, a spouse may say, "I feel so hopeless. I just smack him now to show him he can't pretend I'm not here. He can't wipe out my hurt just like that."

3. The partner, supported by the therapist, begins to hear and understand the significance of the injurious event and to understand it in attachment terms as a reflection of his or her importance to the injured spouse, rather than as a reflection of his or her personal inadequacies or insensitivity. This partner then acknowledges the injured partner's pain and suffering and elaborates on how the event evolved for him or her.

4. The injured partner then tentatively moves toward a more integrated and complete articulation of the injury and expresses grief at the loss involved in it, and fear concerning the specific loss of the attachment bond. This partner allows the other to witness his or her vulnerability.

5. The other spouse becomes more emotionally engaged and acknowledges responsibility for his or her part in the attachment injury and expresses empathy, regret, and/or remorse.

6. The injured spouse then risks asking for the comfort and caring from the partner that were unavailable at the time of the injurious event.

7. The other spouse responds in a caring manner that acts as an antidote to the traumatic experience of the original injury. The partners are then able to construct together a new narrative of the event. This narrative is ordered and includes, for the injured spouse, a clear and acceptable sense of how the other came to respond in such a distressing manner during the event.

Once the attachment injury is resolved, the therapist can more effectively foster the growth of trust and the beginning of positive cycles of bonding and connection. The couple can then complete change events, such as a softening, whereby the more blaming spouse can confide his or her attachment needs and the other can respond (Johnson, 1996). This process defines the relationship as a safe haven, fostering the resolution of other difficulties and pragmatic problems.

The concept of attachment injuries as relationship traumas has important implications for both clinician and clients. This perspective may explain why some couples have more difficulty responding to therapy. Such events must be addressed and resolved to prevent relapse after therapy. The identification of these events also allows for the formulation of a systematic set of interventions for their resolution. Moreover, the delineation of such specific problems and tasks in therapy facilitates inquiry into pivotal factors in the change process. We can then learn to map out the personal and relational factors that predict partners' becoming "stuck" in such injuries and how such injuries may be resolved in therapy. Relational factors, such as the rigidity of negative interactional cycles and the existence of some form of safe emotional engagement and commitment to the relationship, may be critical, as may personal factors such as previous experiences of betrayal (e.g., sexual abuse in childhood tends to make issues of trust and dependency particularly problematic) and the nature of working models of the self and the other. In general, those who have a more secure attachment style seem to cope better with episodes of trust violation in their relationships (Mikulincer, 1998).

For the couples who come to therapy, addressing the task of resolving relational traumas has potential to play a key role in creating or restoring the security of their emotional attachment. This attachment, which is "the primary protection against feelings of helplessness and meaningless" (McFarlane & van der Kolk, 1996, p. 24), is a potent factor in creating resilience both in individual partners and in long-term relationships.

Chapter 11

Therapists Who Deal with Dragons

*T*herapists who stand with their clients to deal with the dragon also feel the heat of the dragon's fire and the frustrations of the battle their clients are fighting. From the beginning, they need to believe that their struggle to understand, to support, and to guide can significantly impact the couple's distressed relationship and a partner's battle with chronic fear and helplessness. More than this, therapists have to believe that the help they offer matters and that *they can make a crucial difference*. Can couple therapy for trauma survivors and their partners truly make such a difference?

We know that if we do not pay attention to and actively treat the attachment relationships of those struggling with posttraumatic stress disorder (PTSD), these relationships most often become part of the problem. Relationship distress then adds to the burden of the survivor and often impedes individual healing. Criticism expressed by attachment figures has been shown to undermine the treatment of trauma in individual therapy (Tarrier, Sommerfield, & Pilgrim, 1999). It also makes sense that if the changes made by an individual in any therapy are to endure, it is often necessary for those changes to occur in and be supported by the natural environment (Gurman, 2001). If therapists who work with trauma survivors and their partners also understand the power of positive attachment to actively heal the wounds of trauma, as perhaps nothing else can, they can have a sense of purpose that helps

them withstand the difficulties of attempting to shape caring and connection out of terror, alienation, and hopelessness. Research clearly tells
us that being able to create a satisfying relationship with a partner enables people to cope positively with past difficulties and traumas and
ameliorates the impact of, for example, institutionalization or bereavement in childhood (Parker & Hadzi-Pavlovic, 1984; Rutter & Quinton,
1984). Study after study tells us that the quality of our most intimate
emotionally charged relationships are deciding factors in how physically and mentally resilient we can become.

The field of psychotherapy has always recognized that the relationship with the therapist offers an opportunity for healing in and of itself,
apart from any insights or other curative factors the process of therapy
may offer. Trauma therapists have been particularly aware that the relationship with the therapist, and the corrective emotional experience
that such a relationship offers, is particularly crucial for trauma survivors. The argument outlined in this book is that helping survivors create healing relationships with the primary attachment figures in their
lives is often at least as important for long-term health as being able to
create a healing relationship with a therapist in individual therapy, particularly once the trauma has been named and confronted, whether in
individual therapy or by some other means. Individual and couple therapy each offer a crucial piece of the puzzle of how to live a full life in
the shadow of the dragon.

It may be argued that until recently couple therapy was not sufficiently systematic or sophisticated to play such a role. At this point,
however, couple therapy has an empirical base for understanding relationship distress and tested, systematic interventions for relieving such
distress. It is significant that both empirically validated interventions—
cognitive-behavioral couple therapy and emotionally focused couple
therapy (EFT)—are supported by data showing that they are effective in
helping partners, not just with relationship distress, but also with depression, and both are now used in clinical practice with the survivors
of trauma (Compton & Follette, 1998; Johnson & Williams Keeler,
1998).

If couple therapy is to take its place as a significant and often crucial element in the treatment of trauma, it is important to note the particular difficulties to be faced in helping survivors to repair their relationships and create bonds that heal.

First, couples who are dealing with trauma are often more distressed than those who are not. They tend to be caught in particularly

absorbing states of negative affect and display intensely compelling and repetitive cycles of defense, distance, and distrust. Herman (1992) has noted, "The core experiences of psychological trauma are disempowerment and disconnection from others" (p. 133). Helping a survivor and his or her spouse create a secure sense of connection is more challenging and requires more support from the therapist than dealing with less intense forms of relationship distress. The therapy process is often slower with traumatized couples, and the therapist has to "slice it thinner." A client once remarked, "You go slow and we repeat steps, and sometimes, when I can't step at all, you stop and make the step smaller. Or you just get me to talk about how I can't make the step right now and what that's about. Sometimes you've even made it okay for me to just stay where I am and weep. This is important."

Emotional storms and crises, and improvements followed by relapses, are inevitable as each partner faces new risks and finds them daunting. These crises certainly involve the survivor's responses to walking in the foreign land of trust and safe dependency. Yet it is important to note that the other partner has often been secondarily traumatized, not only by being a witness to the terrors of the fight with the dragon and vicariously feeling the heat of the dragon's breath, but also by living with the PTSD symptoms of the survivor, such as unpredictable irritability and rage (Catherall, 1992; Nelson & Wampler, 2000). Thus, this partner's response must be taken into account as well.

Second, in treating traumatized couples the therapist has to address ways of dealing with terror that have themselves become particularly problematic, such as not eating, cutting one's body, or other forms of self-injury. Other professionals, particularly the survivor's individual therapist, if he or she has one, can be helpful here. It is important that the couple therapist liaise with other therapists and coordinate treatment efforts with them. The therapist must always be aware of emotional risk and take extra care to set up safety nets, such as contingency plans for moments of despair or panic. The therapist must be sure, as mentioned earlier, to make the steps of change as small as necessary, especially when setting interactional tasks that involve any kind of emotional risk. Emotions have to be contained as well as heightened. Traumatized partners have to be soothed and affirmed more than nontraumatized partners, and their defenses validated and respected to a greater degree. For many of these partners, survival itself has been an extreme and heroic feat. The fact that such partners are attempting to create a loving relationship, which some may never have experienced, is a tribute to the human spirit and to the power of the human need for connection with and comfort from significant others. Bowlby (1969, 1988) believed that attachment needs and longings are wired in by thousands of years of evolution. This perspective goes a long way toward explaining why those who have been so wounded in close relationships, such as survivors of childhood sexual abuse (CSA), are still willing to struggle with their fears in the hope of making such a connection.

Third, less can be assumed about the destination of the therapy journey with traumatized couples than about that of others. The therapist has to be extremely careful to support the couple in creating their own idiosyncratic goals. In particular, incest survivors and their partners usually have to craft their own detailed concept of pleasurable touch and safe sexuality to a much greater extent than nontraumatized couples. At moments of physical closeness, the exquisite nuances of how the self is defined in interactions with attachment figures become apparent. The fear of being seen or exposed and the automatic triggering of shame and self-condemnation are endemic in these survivors. The therapist must be flexible and comfortable in switching between levels of intervention, from structuring couple interactions, to exploring how the self is structured and supporting the taking of new risks, to helping partners formulate ways to minimize the threat involved in activities that other couples find simply rewarding, such as hugging and touching.

The pivotal challenge for the therapist here, however, is the creation of a particular kind of alliance, an alliance in which the therapist can attune to each partner with particular sensitivity. The essence of this alliance is that the therapist is always learning from his or her clients and is open to discovering how each partner experiences the moment-to-moment dance of connection and disconnection. The alliance is, at least at first, often more fragile and requires more monitoring than with other couples. It also requires more intense collaboration and a greater willingness to be transparent on the part of the therapist. The most intense battles with the dragon usually take place in individual therapy, and issues such as the vicarious traumatization of the therapist, although still pertinent, may be less compelling for the couple therapist as compared with the individual therapist. However, the couple therapist has a particularly complex task. He or she has to create a positive collaborative alliance with each partner and slowly structure the therapy process to create a secure healing bond between the two partners. The next section considers, in greater detail, the therapist's role in the treatment of trauma.

THE ROLE OF THE THERAPIST

It has long been recognized that trauma is contagious and that working with those who have been traumatized can be extremely stressful. Some of the sources of such stress, which therapists identified in my hospital clinic, are echoed in the literature (Herman, 1992; Pearlman & Saakvitne, 1995). These are identified in the following paragraphs.

1. In witnessing a client's trauma and identifying with his or her pain, the therapist has to deal with the difficult feelings of sadness, rage, despair, and terror. The therapist must be able to stay grounded and to regulate, process, and integrate difficult emotional material in order to stay engaged with the survivor and validate this person's experience. For clients, seeing the therapist weep for their pain, or become angry at their betrayal, may be powerfully validating . It can also be a revelation, inasmuch as some clients cannot weep or rage for themselves. However, the therapist must draw a line between being available and responsive to the client's experience and maintaining the ability to step back and direct the session in the client's interests. In order to offer clients a safe environment, the therapists must be able to regulate his or her own affect.

2. Sometimes when we weep for others, we suddenly find that it is also ourselves we are weeping for. In the process of the therapist's identifying with clients, therapy may touch and potentially crystallize the griefs, disappointments, and fears in the therapist's own life. Vicarious traumatization, defined as "the transformation in the inner experience of the therapist that comes about as a result of empathic engagement with a client's traumatic material" (Pearlman & Saakvitne, 1995, p. 31), is an occupational hazard. For couple therapists, the process of therapy may bring their own attachment issues to the fore. This can occur in all couple therapy, but the poignancy and emotional intensity of the process with traumatized couples is more likely to exacerbate this process.

3. Connecting with the helplessness of the survivor, and sometimes of the secondarily traumatized spouse, can be overwhelming for the therapist. Being a witness to cruelty and evil and to human vulnerability can be an existential challenge to the therapist's sense of control, security, and meaning in his or her own life. The therapist's philosophical framework for making meaning of the human condition must expand to deal with the experiences related by survivors in therapy. As Davis

and Frawley (1991) point out, to work with survivors, we have to be able to withstand our clients' despair and the fact that we cannot always alleviate their suffering.

4. The rawness and immensity of people's pain can be intimidating for the therapist who wants to "rescue" the survivor, stop the hurt, or find quick solutions when the echoes of trauma take over the couple's dance. The therapist may then struggle with professional identity issues and begin to lose confidence in the process of therapy and the client's ability to heal. A novice therapist once remarked, "This client has no reason on earth to ever trust another human being. There is no room for error—by me or by her spouse. I don't know whether anyone can help her." At such times it is useful for the therapist to hold the perspective that problem behaviors are creative adaptations to impossible situations, rather than pathological responses that doom clients or inevitably severely limit their growth and the quality of their relationships. If we do not respect our clients' defenses, even when they threaten our sense of competence as therapists, we undermine the therapy session as a safe haven and secure base for growth and new learning. A patient, validating stance is harder to maintain, however, when clients "refuse" to validate us by responding to our interventions the way we think they should. It is also useful, in a task-oriented environment, where there is increasing pressure to make therapy efficient and goal directed, to remember that whether therapists are working with individuals, couples, or families, sometimes the only "solution" is to be with our clients and offer them comfort and connection. A secure base is the first stage on the path to change.

5. A survivor's ambivalence about trusting the therapist, and exquisite sensitivity to any lack of attunement or judgment on the part of the therapist, puts additional pressure on that therapist to constantly track how that client is experiencing the session and responding to interventions. A traumatized client may view the therapist's sad facial expression, after that client's revelation of a particularly painful event, as proof of his or her own toxicity. It is hoped that such a response would be picked up by the therapist and addressed. The couple therapist does not usually have to deal with the issue of transference in the same way as an individual therapist. The other partner, rather than the therapist, may at times be responded to as if he or she were a past and often traumatizing attachment figure. However, the level of emotional engagement, with his or her own and both clients' experiences, can still become exhausting.

SELF-CARE FOR THE THERAPIST

Clear conceptual models and maps of the overlapping territories of trauma and attachment relationships have obvious value in helping therapists to formulate key issues and goals for intervention and to choose a set of specific interventions in which they can have confidence. Such models and maps are essential for therapists helping clients deal with the complexities of trauma. Attachment theory offers the therapist who works with traumatized couples a theory of love and relatedness that provides a clear focus for interventions and so makes the complex task facing the therapist much more manageable. The therapist also needs a model of intervention that fits, not only with his or her own personality, but also with the problem at hand. For a model to be appropriate in addressing trauma, it must be one that takes account of the fact that intense emotion is a pivotal part of traumatic stress. Such models of intervention should also be explicitly collaborative. Collaborative approaches are not only more respectful of clients (especially crucial in the alliance with trauma survivors), but also less stressful for the therapist. In such models, there is explicit permission for the therapist to continually learn from his or her clients, rather than to be an expert who has all the answers. Given that the therapist seeks out and constructs an understanding of close relationships and traumatic experience and how they interconnect, and that he or she finds a model of intervention that provides a clear direction and fosters a collaborative relationship with clients, what else is necessary for therapists who wish to help traumatized couples?

First, if we are to help our clients create a secure base for learning, it is essential to have one ourselves. A supportive group of colleagues with whom one can share dilemmas and difficulties is essential. Consultation with such colleagues can be invaluable when we loose our way or become discouraged. Such consultation also helps the therapist to keep the roles, tasks, structure, and boundaries of therapy clear (Perlman & Saakvitne, 1995).

Isolation is hazardous for therapists as well as for clients. Our best protection against vicarious traumatization is a safe haven where we can admit our mistakes, confront our uncertainties, and explore our limitations. The client responses that seem to create most anxiety in therapists are dissociation and suicidal threats or gestures. For survivors, such responses are often the only "escape routes" from an unbearable reality and offer a sense of control. For the therapist, however, such responses often create a sense of loss of control. Consultation with colleagues can help therapists deal with their own dismay and anxiety, so that they do not feel overwhelmed and lose hope at the very moment their clients need them most.

It is almost a cliché in the therapy literature to speak of how important it is for the therapist to be aware of his or her own personal and professional triggers and to avoid being swept up in countertransference reactions. Couple and family therapy have perhaps focused less on this issue, deriving as they do from a systemic orientation. Even this orientation, however, which focuses on how the self of each of the dancers is constantly defined by the nature of the dance, encourages us to be aware that the way we are with clients, not just what we do, is a powerful communicative act that elicits particular responses from those clients. For us, as couple therapists, it is important to be aware of our own attachment beliefs and vulnerabilities and how they can make it difficult for us to attune to particular clients and particular experiences or to be generally empathic. In a society that defines dependency needs in adults as regressive, therapists may have to struggle to accept their own dependency needs. Only then can they consistently validate these needs in their clients and avoid being swept up in the clients' own distrust of such needs, which they may see as proof of their weakness or inadequacy. This negative view of dependency is supported by the dominant Western culture. It is not accidental that Bowlby was branded as a "heretic" by his colleagues. Attachment theory challenges the image of the rugged self-sufficient individual often associated with health and maturity in our society. For example, the couple and family therapy field has, for years, accepted the idea that adolescents have to rebel and "separate" from their parents in order to "individuate." Encouraging the expression of dependency can be viewed as encouraging regression and immaturity. In fact, in my experience and in the theoretical framework of attachment, differentiation and autonomy go hand in hand with connectedness to others.

A humanistic approach, such as that advocated in this book, allows for the disciplined disclosure of the therapist's personal reactions and responses during the therapy session. Such disclosure can be in the interest of the alliance in that it demonstrates the therapist's genuineness and willingness to be seen. Trauma survivors, being exquisitely attuned as they are to the dangers of contact with others, particularly require genuineness from their therapists. Genuineness and openness are also in the interest of the therapist, as they can help the therapist deal with his or her own emotions, such as frustration or confusion. Sharing process dilemmas with the client can be empowering, as long as the therapist does not place the responsibility for leadership on the client. For example, when both partners of a couple are survivors (Matsakis, 1994), there may be times when it is difficult to decide who is to go first in terms of confiding or risking in general. The therapist can share this dilemma.

The therapist's disclosure of personal responses can also be an active intervention, offering clients an alternative perspective on their experiences. As suggested previously, it may be particularly useful for the therapist to be able to express his or her emotional response (such as sadness) to the hurt and fear these clients must deal with, especially when they feel ashamed and/or are unable to have compassion for their own pain and vulnerability. Receiving a compassionate response from the therapist can also be a stepping stone to the ability to receive and trust a similar response from a spouse (see the excerpt in Johnson & Williams Keeler, 1998, pp. 34–36). Many survivors also constantly battle with defining what is real or true. It is useful for the therapist to be able to share his or her sense of reality at particular moments. Clients can then use this as a touchstone and so begin to feel their way through the dark. It is important to note here that therapist disclosure is in the service of clients. If there are personal issues that interfere with the therapist's ability to be fully present in the session to any real extent, these issues should be shared and dealt with in consultation with colleagues or in formal supervision with a mentor. Perhaps the issue of dealing with how the voices of our clients echo in our own hearts, and sometimes interfere with our ability to listen with sensitivity, can be summed up by the words of Pearlman and Saakvitne (1995), who state that in individual therapy "we are the tools of our trade" (p. 185). As these authors suggest, we must know our own issues and limits so as to be able to be responsive to the needs of our clients. This is equally true in couple and family therapy, where the emphasis is often on brief interventions to shift interactions. Couple therapy with trauma survivors may indeed be briefer and more circumscribed than individual therapy; however, the person of the therapist and how his or her personhood is expressed still constitute the basic context that gives meaning to any intervention.

The therapist who wishes to help traumatized couples must also be aware of his or her own limits. Dragons call forth heroes. It is important not to try to be one. My own clinical experience suggests that having more than a third of one's clients dealing with relationship distress and the shadow of the dragon at any one time renders one vulnerable to burnout. It is also important not to mix the roles of couple therapist and individual therapist. Although I have done this in the past, it is a complicated undertaking and experience has taught me that keeping the *relationship* as the client is both simpler and more productive. Relinquishing the role of hero therapist fosters a certain humility and acceptance of one's own mistakes. It fosters an attitude that echoes John Bowlby's sentiments in the dedication in his 1973 book, where he thanks his clients who "have labored so hard to educate me."

THE REWARDS OF WORKING WITH TRAUMATIZED COUPLES

Given the challenges of this work, it is important also to note the rewards.

One of the great rewards of working with couples who are struggling to forge a loving relationship in the shadow of traumatic experience is that times of crisis and suffering are also opportunities for great learning and growth, for the couple and for the therapist. We learn more about how to be human and about our own humanity by being with those who have faced the darkness and found ways to survive and fight on. We understand ourselves better and become better integrated when we help others engage with their experiences, integrate elements of self, and integrate a new sense of self into a relationship with another. One way of conceptualizing this is to consider the engagement with the experience of others as a way of expanding the self (Arons & Arons, 1997). When we share others' choices and struggles, it is as if we get to live more than one life.

The opportunity for learning in the professional arena offered by this work is vast. The primary personal reason I work with traumatized couples is that I am caught and fascinated by the process. Precisely because traumatized couples have extreme cycles of distress, powerful emotions, and compelling needs and fears, they can teach us about the nature of human attachments, the steps in the change process, and the different ways to potentiate this process. This learning can then enrich the therapist's work with all couples and families, traumatized or not.

The second great reward is the potential to have a tremendous positive impact on our clients' lives. There are a number of interventions that can help trauma survivors mitigate their intrusive symptoms. Yet it seems that working with survivors to enable them to connect with key attachment figures in a more trusting way, and so to lessen the need for strategies such as numbing, is at the heart of healing the wounds of trauma. The essence of healing the "violation of human connection" (Herman, 1992, p. 54), which is the key element in many traumas, is the creation of a secure bond with a significant other. This other can then provide a safe haven and a secure base for lifelong learning and growth. It is interesting to note that studies of prisoner relationships in the Nazi death camps found that the vast majority of survivors had become part of a "stable pair" and thus concluded that in situations of chronic danger, the pair rather than the individual is the basic unit of survival (Dimsdale, 1980; Levi, 1961). It may also be that couple therapy as a modality has a unique contribution to make to the treatment of trauma in that it can address issues that are difficult to address elsewhere. For example, shame has been found to mediate the contribution of early victimization to later adult psychological problems and diagnoses (Andrews, Brewin, Rose, & Kirk, 2000). Traditional individual therapy techniques (e.g., exposure), however, may even exacerbate symptoms such as shame (Rothbaum & Foa, 1996). The affirmation of a loved one in couple therapy, on the other hand, seems to positively impact shame and self-disgust. In general, couple therapists have the potential to help their clients create a more loving relationship, and there is no better resource to help us navigate through life or to build resilient families (Ornish, 1998). For the survivor, such a relationship may be the *only* context in which the dragon can be dealt with—and defeated. Moreover, couple therapy allows survivors to struggle with the central issue of basic trust for their fellow humans.

A positive attachment relationship is also the best arena for the fostering of an acceptable sense of self in the survivor. In this relationship the sense of self, often seen as toxic, broken, contaminated by shame, and almost certainly unentitled to love and caring, can be redefined. Those of us who are able to form a secure sense of connection with others not only have a more positive view of ourselves, we seem to have a more balanced, complex, and coherent self-structure (Mikulincer, 1995). A secure connection with others allows us to create an integrated sense of self and to tolerate and cope with our own vulnerabilities. Some traumatized couples will be able to create a relationship that fosters a positive sense of self on their own, or with the aid of self-help resources (Matsakis, 1997). Many, however, will need the guidance of a couple therapist.

Finally, we know that depression and posttraumatic stress are the mental health problems that most often accompany and are exacerbated by marital distress (Whisman, 1999). Learning to work with such distressed couples is crucial to the growth of the field of couple therapy as a whole. A focus on trauma and its impact is changing the way we understand our clients' problems in general and the nature of their distress (Pearlman & Saakvitne, 1995). This change in perception moves the field of psychotherapy from models that stress illness, personal deficits, and symptoms, toward models that emphasize how people have learned to adapt and survive in specific difficult contexts and have not been able to respond to the demands of new and different contexts. There has also been a shift away from the model in which expert therapists guide deficient clients to a model in which the client's problems are treated in a collaborative alliance with a therapist who is a respectful consultant in the change process. A recognition of the impact of traumatic experience and its aftermath moves the general field of psychotherapy closer to a systemic focus on events in interpersonal contexts and how they impact the way clients construe themselves and the world. To deal with trauma, the therapist has to address the specific ways in which both intrapsychic and outer relational realities continually shape each other. As the field of couple therapy integrates a focus on emotional experience, regulation, and communication, including the echoes of trauma, and is able to work with how emotional responses shape key interactions, couple therapy can begin to take its place as a major therapeutic modality—one that addresses both self and system and offers a specific and unique agent of healing, the creation of a secure attachment bond. Such a bond offers us a safe haven and a secure base—a place to stand and face dragons.

References

Abrams Spring, J. A. (1997). *After the affair: Healing the pain and rebuilding trust when a partner has been unfaithful.* New York: Harper Perennial.

Ainsworth, M. D. S., Blehar, M. C., Waters, E., & Wall, S. (1978). *Patterns of attachment: A psychological study of the strange situation.* Hillsdale, NJ: Erlbaum.

Alexander, P. C. (1993). Application of attachment theory to the study of sexual abuse. *Journal of Consulting and Clinical Psychology, 60,* 185–195

Alexander, P. C., & Andersen, C. L. (1994). An attachment approach to psychotherapy with the incest survivor. *Psychotherapy, 31,* 665–675.

Alexander, P. C., Neimeyer, R. A., Follette, V. M., Moore, M. M., & Harter, S. (1989). A comparison of group treatments of women sexually abused as children. *Journal of Consulting and Clinical Psychology, 57,* 479–483.

American Psychiatric Association. (1994). *Diagnostic and statistical manual of mental disorders* (4th ed.). Washington, DC: Author.

Anders, S. L., & Tucker, J. S. (2000). Adult attachment style, interpersonal communication competence and social support. *Personal Relationships, 7,* 379–389.

Anderson, H. (1997). *Conversation, language and possibilities.* New York: Basic Books.

Anderson, P., Beach, S. R. H., & Kaslow, N. J. (1999). Marital discord and depression: The potential of attachment theory to guide intervention. In T. Joiner & J. C. Coyne (Eds.), *The interactional nature of depression* (pp. 271–298). Washington, DC: APA Press.

Andrews, B. (1995). Bodily shame as a mediator between abusive experiences and depression. *Journal of Abnormal Psychology, 104,* 277–285.

Andrews, B., Brewin, C. R., Rose, S., & Kirk, M. (2000). Predicting PTSD symptoms in victims of violent crime: The role of shame, anger and childhood abuse. *Journal of Abnormal Psychology, 109,* 69–73.

Arons, A., & Arons, E. N. (1997). Self-expansion motivation and including the other in the self. In W. Ickes & S. Duck (Eds.), *Handbook of personal relationships* (2nd ed., Vol. 1, pp. 251–270). London: Wiley.

Atkinson, L. (1997). Attachment and psychopathology: From laboratory to clinic. In L. Atkinson & K. J. Zucker (Eds.), *Attachment and psychopathology* (pp. 3–16). New York: Guilford Press.

Badgely, R., Allard, H., McCormick, N., Proudfoot, P., Fortin, D., Oglivie, D., Rae-Grant, Q., Gelinas, P., Penin, L., & Sutherland, S. Committee on Sexual Offences Against Children and Youth (1984). *Sexual offences against children* (Vol. 1). Ottawa, Ontario, Canada: Canadian Government Publishing Centre.

Barlow, D. H., O'Brien, G. T., & Last, C. G. (1984). The treatment of agoraphobia. *Behavior Therapy, 15,* 41–58.

Barnes, M. F. (1998). Understanding the secondary traumatic stress of parents. In C. R. Figley (Ed.), *Burnout in families: The systemic costs of caring* (pp. 75–89). Boca Raton, FL: CRC Press.

Bartholome, K., & Horowitz, L. (1991). Attachment styles among young adults. *Journal of Personality and Social Psychology, 61,* 226–244.

Bartholomew, K., & Perlman, D. (1994). *Attachment processes in adulthood.* London: Jessica Kingsley.

Bateson, G. (1972). *Steps to an ecology of mind.* New York: Chandler.

Baucom, D., Shoham, V., Mueser, K., Daiuto, A., & Stickle, T. (1998). Empirically supported couple and family interventions for marital distress and adult mental health problems. *Journal of Consulting and Clinical Psychology, 66,* 53–88.

Berger, P., & Luckmann, T. (1979). *The social construction of reality.* Harmondsworth, UK: Penguin Books.

Bernstein, E. M., & Putnam, F. W. (1986). Development, reliability, and validity of a dissociation scale. *Journal of Nervous and Mental Disease, 174,* 727–735.

Blake, D. D. (1993). Treatment outcome on post traumatic stress disorder. *CP Clinical Newsletter, 3,* 14–17.

Blake, D. D., Weathers, F. W., Nagy, L. M., Kaloupek, D. G., Klauminger, G., Charney, D. S., & Keane, T. M. (1990). A clinician rating scale for assessing current lifetime PTSD: The CAPS 1. *The Behavior Therapist, 18,* 181–188.

Bograd, M., & Mederos, F. (1999). Battering and couples therapy: Universal screening and selection of treatment modality. *Journal of Marital and Family Therapy, 25,* 291–312.

Bowlby, J. (1949). The study and reduction of group tensions in the family. *Human Relations, 2,* 123–128.

Bowlby, J. (1969). *Attachment and loss: Vol 1. Attachment.* New York: Basic Books.

Bowlby, J. (1973). *Attachment and loss: Vol II. Separation.* New York: Basic Books.

Bowlby, J. (1980). *Attachment and loss: Vol III. Loss.* New York: Basic Books.

Bowlby, J. (1988). *A secure base.* New York. Basic Books.

Breslau, N., Davis, G. C. D., Andreski, P., & Peterson, E. (1991). Traumatic events and posttraumatic stress disorder in an urban population of young adults. *Archives of General Psychiatry, 48,* 218–222.

Bretherton, I., & Munholland, K. A. (1999). Internal working models in attachment relationships: A construct revisited. In J. Cassidy & P. R. Shaver (Eds.), *Handbook of attachment: Theory, research, and clinical applications* (pp. 89–114). New York: Guilford Press.

Breuer, J., & Freud, S. (1956). *Studies on hysteria, Vol. 2* (J. S. Strachey, Trans.). London: Hogarth Press.

Brom, D., & Kleber, R. J. (1989). Brief psychotherapy for post traumatic stress disorders. *Journal of Consulting and Clinical Psychology, 57,* 607–612.

Burman, B., & Margolin, G. (1992). Analysis of the association between marital relationships and health problems: An interactional perspective. *Psychological Bulletin, 112,* 39–63.

Busby, D. M., Christensen, C., Crane, D. R., & Larsen, J. H. (1995). A revision of the dyadic adjustment scale for use with distressed and non-distressed couples: Construct hierarchy and multidimensional scales. *Journal of Marital and Family Therapy, 21,* 289–308.

Carney, R. M., Rich, M. W., Freedland, K. E., Saini, J., TeVelde, A., Simeone, C., & Clark, K. (1988). Major depressive disorder predicts cardiac events in patients with coronary heart disease. *Psychosomatic Medicine, 50,* 603–609.

Carroll, E. M., Foy, D. W., Cannon, B. J., & Zwler, G. (1991). Assessment issues involving families of trauma victims. *Journal of Traumatic Stress, 4,* 25–35.

Cassidy, J., & Shaver, P. R. (Eds.). (1999). *Handbook of attachment: Theory, research, and clinical applications.* New York: Guilford Press.

Catherall, D. R. (1992). *Back from the brink: A family guide to overcoming traumatic stress.* New York: Bantam.

Cerny, J. A., Barlow, D. H., Craske, M. G., & Himadi, W. G. (1987). Couples treatment of agoraphobia: A two year follow-up. *Behavior Therapy, 18,* 401–415.

Chu, J. A. (1992). The revictimization of adult women with histories of childhood abuse. *Journal of Psychotherapy Practice and Research, 1,* 259–269.

Chu, J. A. (1998). *Rebuilding shattered lives: The responsible treatment of complex post-traumatic and dissociative disorders.* New York: Wiley.

Coble, H. M., Gantt, D. L., & Mallinckrodt, B. (1996). Attachment, social competency, and the capacity to use social support. In G. Pierce & B. R. Sarason (Eds.), *Handbook of social support and the family* (pp. 141–172). New York: Plenum Press.

Coffey, P., Leitenberg, H., Henning, K., & Turner, T. (1996). Mediators of the long term impact of child sexual abuse: Perceived stigma, betrayal, powerlessness and self-blame. *Child Abuse and Neglect, 20,* 447–455.

Cohn, D., Silver, D., Cowan, C., Cowan, P., & Pearson, J. (1992). Working models of childhood attachment and couple relationships. *Journal of Family Issues, 13,* 432–449.

Collins, N., & Read, S. (1994). Cognitive representations of attachment: The structure and function of working models. In K. Bartholomew & D. Perlman (Eds.), *Attachment processes in adulthood* (pp. 53–92). London: Jessica Kingsley.

Compton, J. S., & Follette, V. M. (1998). Couples surviving trauma: Issues and interventions. In V. M. Follette, J. I. Ruzek, & F. R. Abueg (Eds.), *Cognitive-behavioral therapies for trauma* (pp. 321–352). New York: Guilford Press.

Coop Gordon, K., Baucom, D. S., & Snyder, D. (2000). The use of forgiveness in marital therapy. In M. E. McCullough, K. I. Pargament, & C. E. Thoresen (Eds.), *Forgiveness: Theory, research, and practice* (pp. 203–227). New York: Guilford Press.

Cordova, M. J., Andrykowski, M. A., Kenady, D. E., McGrath, P. C., Sloan, D. A., & Redd, W. H. (1995). Frequency and correlates of posttraumatic stress disorder-like symptoms after the treatment of breast cancer. *Journal of Consulting and Clinical Psychology, 63,* 981–986.

Courtois, C. (1988). *Healing the incest wound: Adult survivors in therapy.* New York: Norton.

Craske, M. G., & Zoellner, L. A. (1995). Anxiety disorders: The role of marital therapy. In N. S. Jacobson & A. S. Gurman (Eds.), *Clinical handbook of couple therapy* (pp. 394–410). New York: Guilford Press.

Davila, J., Karney, B., & Bradbury, T. N. (1999). Attachment change processes in the early years of marriage. *Journal of Personality and Social Psychology, 76,* 783–802.

Davis, J. M., & Frawley, M. G. (1991). Dissociative processes and countertransference paradigms in the psychoanalytically oriented treatment of adult survivors of childhood sexual abuse. *Psychoanalytic Dialogues, 2,* 5–36.

Derogatis, L. R. (1977). *The SCL-90 Manual: Vol I. Scoring, administration and procedures for the SCL-90.* Baltimore: Johns Hopkins University School of Medicine.

Dimsdale, J. E. (1980). *Survivors, victims and perpetrators: Essays on the Nazi holocaust.* New York: Hemisphere.

Donovan, J. M. (1999). Short-term couple therapy and the principles of brief treatment. In J. M Donovan (Ed.), *Short-term couple therapy* (pp. 1–9). New York: Guilford Press.

Dozier, M., & Kobak, R. (1992). Psychophysiology in adolescent attachment interviews: Converging evidence for deactivating strategies. *Child Development, 63,* 1473–1480.

Duncan, B., Miller, S., & Sparks, J. (2000, April). Exposing the myth makers. *Family Therapy Networker,* pp. 24–33, 52–53.

Dutton, D. G. (1995). *The batterer: A psychological profile.* New York: Basic Books.

Ekman, P., & Friesen, W. (1975). *Unmasking the face.* Englewood Cliffs, NJ: Prentice-Hall.

Enright, R. D., & Fitzgibbons, R. P (2000). *Helping clients forgive: An empirical guide for resolving anger and restoring hope.* Washington, DC: APA Press.

Erdman, P., & Caffery, T. (Eds.). (in press). *Attachment and family systems: Conceptual, empirical and therapeutic relatedness.* Philadelphia: Brunner-Routledge.

Figley, C. R. (1989). *Healing traumatized families.* San Francisco: Jossey-Bass.

Figley, C. R. (1995). Compassion fatigue as secondary traumatic stress disorder: An overview. In C. R. Figley (Ed.), *Compassion fatigue: Coping with secondary traumatic stress disorder in those who treat the traumatized* (pp. 1–21). New York: Brunner/Mazel.

Finkelhor, D. (1984). *Child sexual abuse: New theory and research.* New York: Free Press.

Finkelhor, D., & Browne, A. (1984). The traumatic impact of child sexual abuse: A conceptualization. *American Journal of Orthopsychiatry, 55,* 530–541.

Flanigan, B. (1992). *Forgiving the unforgivable.* New York: Macmillian.

Foa, E. B., Hearst-Ikeda, D., & Perry, K. J. (1995). Evaluation of a brief behavioral program for the prevention of chronic PTSD in recent assault victims. *Journal of Consulting and Clinical Psychology, 63,* 948–955.

Foa, E. B., & Riggs, D. S. (1993). Post-traumatic stress disorder in rape victims. In

J. Oldam, M. Riba, & A. Tasman (Eds.), *American Psychiatric Press review of psychiatry* (Vol. 12, pp. 273–303). Washington, DC: American Psychiatric Press.

Foa, E. B., Riggs, D. S., Dancu, C. V., & Rothbaum, B. O. (1993). Reliability and validity of a brief instrument for assessing post-traumatic stress disorder. *Journal of Traumatic Stress, 6,* 459–474.

Foa, E. B., & Rothbaum, B. O. (1998). *Treating the trauma of rape: Cognitive-behavioral therapy for PTSD.* New York: Guilford Press.

Follette, V. M., Polusny, M. A., Bechtle, A. E., & Naugle, A. E. (1996). Cumulative trauma: The impact of child sexual abuse, adult sexual assault, and spouse abuse. *Journal of Traumatic Stress, 9,* 25–35.

Fonagy, P., Steele, H., & Steele, M. (1991). Maternal representations of attachment during pregnancy predict the organization of infant–mother attachment at one year of age. *Child Development, 62,* 891–905.

Fonagy, P., Steele, M., Steele, H., Leigh, T., Kennedy, R., Mattoon, G., & Target, M. (1995). Attachment, the reflective self and borderline states. In S. Goldberg, R. Muir, & J. Kerr (Eds.), *Attachment theory: Social developmental and clinical perspectives* (pp. 233–278). Hillsdale, NJ: Analytic Press.

Fonagy, P., & Target, M. (1997). Attachment and reflective function: Their role in self-organization. *Development and Psychopathology, 9,* 679–700.

Fontana, A., Rosenheck, R., & Brett, E. (1992). War zone traumas and posttraumatic stress disorder symptomatology. *Journal of Nervous and Mental Disease, 8,* 748–755.

Fraley, R. C., & Waller, N. G. (1998). Adult attachment patterns: A test of the typological model. In J. A. Simpson & W. S. Rholes (Eds.), *Attachment theory and close relationships* (pp. 77–114). New York: Guilford Press.

Freedman, J., & Combs, G. (1996). *Narrative therapy.* New York: Norton.

Frijda, N. (1986). *The emotions.* New York: Cambridge University Press.

Gendlin, E. T. (1981). *Focusing* (2nd ed.). New York: Bantam Books.

George, C., Kaplan, N., & Main, M. (1984). *Adult Attachment Interview.* Unpublished manuscript, University of California, Berkeley.

Gergen, K. J. (1994). *Realities and relationships.* Cambridge, MA: Harvard University Press.

Gersons, B., & Carlier, I. (1994). Treatment of work related trauma in police officers. In M. Williams & J. Sommer (Eds.), *Handbook of post trauma therapy* (pp. 325–336). Westport, CT: Greenwood Press.

Goleman, D. (1995). *Emotional intelligence.* New York: Bantam Books.

Gottman, J. (1991). Predicting the longitudinal course of marriages. *Journal of Marital and Family Therapy, 17,* 3–7.

Gottman, J. (1994). *What predicts divorce?* Hillsdale, NJ: Erlbaum.

Gottman, J. (1999). *The marriage clinic: A scientifically based marital therapy.* New York: Norton.

Gottman, J., Coan, J., Carrere, S., & Swanson, C. (1998). Predicting marital happiness and stability from newlywed interactions. *Journal of Marriage and the Family, 60,* 5–22.

Greenberg, L. S., & Johnson, S. M. (1988). *Emotionally focused therapy for couples.* New York: Guilford Press.

Greenberg, L. S., Rice, L. N., & Elliott, R. (1993). *Facilitating emotional change: The moment-by-moment process.* New York: Guilford Press.

Gross J. J., & Levenson, R. W. (1993). Emotional suppression: Physiology, self-report and expressive behavior. *Journal of Personality and Social Psychology, 64,* 970–986.

Grossman, F. K., Cook, A. B., Kepkep, S. S., & Koenen, K. C. (1999). *With the phoenix rising: Lessons from ten resilient women who overcame the trauma of childhood sexual abuse.* San Francisco: Jossey-Bass.

Guerney, B. G. (1994). The role of emotion in relationship enhancement marital/family therapy. In S. M. Johnson & L. S. Greenberg (Eds.), *The heart of the matter: Perspectives on emotion in marital therapy* (pp. 124–150). New York: Brunner/Mazel.

Gurman, A. (2001). Brief therapy and family and couple therapy: An essential redundancy. *Clinical Psychology: Science and Practice, 8,* 51–65.

Gurman, A. S., & Lebow, J. (2000). Family and couple therapy. In B. Sadock & H. Kaplan (Eds.), *Comprehensive textbook of psychiatry* (7th ed., pp. 2157–2166). Baltimore: Williams & Wilkins.

Haddock, S., Schindler Zimmerman, T., & MacPhee, D. (2000). The power equity guide: Attending to gender in family therapy. *Journal of Marital and Family Therapy, 26,* 153–170.

Halford, K. W., Scott, J. L., & Smythe, J. (2000). Couples and coping with cancer: Helping each other through the night. In K. B. Schmaling & T. Goldman Sher (Eds.), *The psychology of couples and illness: Theory, research and practice* (pp. 135–170). Washington, DC: APA Press.

Hargrave, T. D., & Sells, J. N. (1997). The development of a forgiveness scale. *Journal of Marital and Family Therapy, 23,* 41–62.

Harvey, M. (1996). An ecological view of psychological trauma and trauma recovery. *Journal of Traumatic Stress, 9,* 3–23.

Hazan, C., & Shaver, P. (1987). Conceptualizing romantic love as an attachment process. *Journal of Personality and Social Psychology, 52,* 511–524.

Hazan, C., & Shaver, P. (1994). Attachment as an organizational framework for research on close relationships: Target article. *Psychological Inquiry, 5,* 1–22.

Helgeson, V. S., & Cohen, S. (1996). Social support and adjustment to cancer: Reconciling descriptive, correlational and intervention research. *Health Psychology, 15,* 135–148.

Hendrix, H. (1988). *Getting the love you want: A guide for couples.* New York: Henry Holt.

Herman, J. L. (1981). *Father–daughter incest.* Cambridge, MA: Harvard University Press.

Herman, J. L. (1992). *Trauma and recovery.* New York: Basic Books.

Herman, J. L. (1993). Complex PTSD: A syndrome in survivors of prolonged and repeated trauma. *Journal of Traumatic Stress, 5,* 377–391.

Himelein, M. J., & McElrath, J. V. (1996). Resilient child sexual abuse survivors: Cognitive coping and illusion. *Child Abuse and Neglect, 20,* 747–758.

Holmes, J. G., Boon, S. D., & Adams, S. (1990). *The Relationship Trust Scale.* Unpublished manuscript, University of Waterloo, Ontario, Canada.

Hooley, J. M. (1990). Expressed emotion and depression. In G. I Keitner (Ed.), *De-*

pression in families: Impact and treatment (pp. 57–83). Washington, DC: American Psychiatric Press.

Horowitz, M. J. (1986). Stress response syndromes: A review of posttraumatic and adjustment disorders. *Hospital and Community Psychiatry, 37,* 241–249.

House, J. S., Landis, K. R., & Umberson, D. (1988). Social relationships and health. *Science, 24,* 540–545.

Izard, C., & Youngstrom, E. A. (1996). The activation and regulation of fear. In D. A. Hope (Ed.), *Nebraska Symposium on Motivation: Vol. 43. Perspectives on anxiety, panic and fear: Current theory and research in motivation* (pp. 1–59). Lincoln: University of Nebraska Press.

Jamison, R. N., & Virts, K. L. (1990). The influence of family support on chronic pain. *Behaviour Research and Therapy, 28,* 283–287.

Johnson, S. M. (1986). Bonds or bargains: Relationship paradigms and their significance for marital therapy. *Journal of Marital and Family Therapy, 12,* 259–267.

Johnson, S. M. (1993). *Healing broken bonds: A marital therapy training video* [Videotape]. (Available from Ottawa Couple & Family Institute, #201, 1869 Carling Avenue, Ottawa, ON, Canada K2A 1E6)

Johnson, S. M. (1996). *The practice of emotionally focused marital therapy: Creating connection.* New York: Brunner/Mazel.

Johnson, S. M. (1997, September). The biology of love. *Family Therapy Networker,* pp. 36–41.

Johnson, S. M. (1998). Listening to the music: Emotion as a natural part of systems theory. *Journal of Systemic Therapies: Special Edition on the Use of Emotions in Couple and Family Therapy, 17,* 1–17.

Johnson, S. M. (1999). Emotionally focused couple therapy: Straight to the heart. In J. M. Donovan (Ed.), *Short-term couple therapy* (pp. 13–42). New York: Guilford Press.

Johnson, S. M. (in press). An antidote to posttraumatic stress disorder: The creation of secure attachment. In L. Atkinson (Ed.), *Applications of attachment.* New York: Erlbaum.

Johnson, S. M., & Best, M. (in press). A systemic approach to restructuring attachment: The EFT model of couple therapy. In P. Erdman & T. Caffery (Eds.), *Attachment and family systems: Conceptual, empirical and therapeutic relatedness.* Philadelphia: Brunner- Routledge.

Johnson, S. M., & Denton, W. (forthcoming). Emotionally focused couple therapy: Creativity connection. In A. S. Gurman & N. S. Jacobson (Eds.), *Clinical handbook of couple therapy* (2nd ed.). New York: Guilford Press.

Johnson, S. M., & Greenberg, L. (1988). Relating process to outcome in marital therapy. *Journal of Marital and Family Therapy, 14,* 175–183.

Johnson, S. M., & Greenberg, L. (1992). Emotionally focused therapy: Restructuring attachment. In S. H. Budman, M. F. Hoyt, & S. Friedman (Eds.), *The first session in brief therapy* (pp. 204–224). New York: Guilford Press.

Johnson, S. M., & Greenberg, L. S. (1994). *The heart of the matter: Perspectives on emotion in marital therapy.* New York: Brunner/Mazel.

Johnson, S. M., Hunsley, J., Greenberg, L., & Schlindler, D. (1999). Emotionally focused couples therapy: Status and challenges. *Clinical Psychology: Science and Practice, 6,* 67–79.

Johnson, S. M., & Lebow, J. (2000). The coming of age of couple therapy: A decade review. *Journal of Marital and Family Therapy, 26,* 23–38.

Johnson, S. M., Makinen, J., & Millikin, J. (2001). Attachment injuries in couple relationships: A new perspective on impasses in couples therapy. *Journal of Marital and Family Therapy, 27,* 145–156.

Johnson, S. M., & Talitman, E. (1997). Predictors of success in emotionally focused marital therapy. *Journal of Marital and Family Therapy, 23,* 135–152.

Johnson, S. M., & Whiffen, V. (1999). Made to measure: Adapting emotionally focused couples therapy to couples attachment styles. In M. Whisman & D. Snyder (Eds.), *Special Edition of Clinical Psychology: Science and Practice, Affective and Developmental Considerations in Couples Therapy, 6,* 366–381.

Johnson, S. M., & Williams Keeler, L. (1998). Creating healing relationships for couples dealing with trauma: The use of emotionally focused therapy. *Journal of Marital and Family Therapy, 24,* 25–40.

Joiner, T., & Coyne, J. C. (Eds.). (1999). *The interactional nature of depression.* Washington, DC: APA Press.

Jordan, J. V., Kaplan, A. G., Miller, J. B., Stiver, I. P., & Surrey, J. L. (1991). *Women's growth in connection: Writings from the Stone Center.* New York: Guilford Press.

Kardiner, A. (1941). *The traumatic neuroses of war.* New York: Hoeber.

Kardiner, A., & Spiegel, H. (1947). *War stress and neurotic illness.* New York: Hoeber.

Karen, R. (1998). *Becoming attached: First relationships and how they shape our capacity to love.* New York: Oxford University Press.

Keane, T. M., Scott, W. O., Chavoya, G. A., Lamparski, D. M., & Fairbank, J. A. (1985). Social support in Vietnam veterans with posttraumatic stress disorder. *Journal of Consulting and Clinical Psychology, 53,* 95–102.

Keesler, R. C., Sonnega, A., Bromet, E., Hughes, M., & Nelson, C. B. (1995). Post traumatic stress disorder in National Comorbidity Survey. *Archives of General Psychiatry, 52,* 1048–1060.

Kennedy-Moore, E., & Watson, J. C. (1999). *Expressing emotion: Myths, realities, and therapeutic strategies.* New York: Guilford Press.

Kiecolt-Glaser, J. K., & Glaser, J. (1995). Measurement of immune response. In S. Cohen, R. Kessler, & L. U. Gordon (Eds.), *Measuring stress: A guide for health and social scientists* (pp. 213–229). New York: Oxford University Press.

Kiecolt-Glaser, J. K., Malarkey, W. B., Chee, M., Newton, T., Cacioppo, J., Mao, H. Y., & Glaser, J. (1993). Negative behavior during marital conflict is associated with immunological down-regulation. *Psychosomatic Medicine, 55,* 395–409.

Kiecolt-Glaser, J. K., Page, G. G., Marucha, P. T., MacCallum, R. C., & Glaser, R. (1998). Psychological influences on surgical recovery. *American Psychologist, 53,* 1209–1218.

Kilpatrick, D. G., Saunders, B. E., Veranen, L. J., Best, C. L., & Van, J. M. (1987). Criminal victimization: Lifetime prevalence and psychological impact. *Crime and Delinquency, 33,* 479–489.

King, D. W., King, L. A., Foy, D. W., & Gudanowski, D. M. (1996). Prewar factors in combat related posttraumatic stress disorder. *Journal of Consulting and Clinical Psychology, 64,* 520–531.

Kobak, R., & Cole, H. (1991). Attachment and meta-monitoring: Implications for adolescent autonomy and psychopathology. In D. Cicchetti & S. Toth (Eds.), *Disorders and dysfunctions of the self* (pp. 267–297). Rochester, NY: University of Rochester Press.

Kobak, R., & Duemmler, S. (1994). Attachment and conversation: A discourse analysis of goal directed partnerships. In K. Bartholomew & D. Perlman (Eds.), *Advances in personal relationships: Vol 5. Attachment processes in adulthood* (pp. 121–149). London: Jessica Kingsley.

Kobak, R., & Hazan, C. (1991). Attachment in marriage: The effects of security and accuracy in working models. *Journal of Personality and Social Psychology, 60,* 861–869.

Kobak, R., & Sceery, A. (1988). Attachment in late adolescence: Working models, affect regulation and representations of self and others. *Child Development, 59,* 135–146.

Krantz, D. S., Contrada, R. J., Hill, R. O., & Friedler, E. (1988). Environmental stress and biobehavioral antecedents of coronary heart disease. *Journal of Consulting and Clinical Psychology, 65,* 333–341.

Kulik, J. A., & Mahler, H. I. (1989). Social support and recovery from surgery. *Health Psychology, 8,* 221–238.

Kulka, R., Schlenger, W., Fairbank, J., Hough, R., Jordan, B., Marmar, C., & Weiss, D. (1990). *Trauma and the Vietnam war generation: Report of findings from the National Vietnam Veterans Readjustment Study.* New York: Brunner/Mazel.

Lamb, W. (1998). *I know this much is true.* New York: Regan Books.

Lang, P. (1979). A bio-informational theory of emotional imagery. *Psychophysiology, 16,* 495–512.

Levi, P. (1961). *Survival in Auschwitz: The Nazi assault on humanity.* New York: Collier.

Litz, B. T., Schlenger, W., Weathers, F., Caddell, J., Fairband, J., & Lavange, L. (1997). Predictors of emotional numbing in posttraumatic stress disorder. *Journal of Traumatic Stress, 10,* 607–618.

Litz, B. T., & Weathers, F. W. (1994). The diagnosis and assessment of post-traumatic stress disorder in adults. In M. B. Williams & J. F. Sommer (Eds.), *Handbook of post-traumatic therapy* (pp. 19–37). Westport, CA: Greenwood Press.

Main, M. (1991). Meta-cognitive knowledge, meta-cognitive monitoring and singular (coherent). vs multiple (incoherent). models of attachment. In J. S. Stevenson-Hinde, C. M. Parkes, & P. Marris (Eds.), *Attachment across the life cycle* (pp. 127–159). London: Routledge.

Main, M., & Hesse, E. (1990). Parents' unresolved traumatic experiences are related to infant disorganized attachment status. In M. Greenberg & D. Cicchetti (Eds.), *Attachment in the preschool years* (pp. 152–176). Chicago: University of Chicago Press.

Main, M., Kaplan, N., & Cassidy, J. (1985). Security in infancy, childhood and adulthood: A move to the level of representation. In I. Bretherton & E. Waters (Eds.), Growing points of attachment theory and research. *Monographs of the Society for Research in Child Development, 50*(1–2, Serial No. 209), 66–106.

Manne, S. L. (1999). Intrusive thoughts and psychological distress among cancer patients: The role of spouse avoidance and criticism. *Journal of Consulting and Clinical Psychology, 67,* 539–546.

Manne, S. L., & Zautra, A. J. (1989). Spouse criticism and support: Their association with coping and psychological adjustment among women with rheumatoid arthritis. *Journal of Personality and Social Psychology, 56,* 608–617.

Manson, S. M. (1997). Cross-cultural and multiethnic assessment of trauma. In J. P. Wilson & T. M. Keane (Eds.), *Assessing psychological trauma and PTSD* (pp. 239–266). New York: Guilford Press.

Matsakis, A. (1994). Dual, triple and quadruple trauma couples: Dynamics and treatment issues. In M. B. Williams & J. F. Sommer (Eds.), *Handbook of post-traumatic therapy* (pp. 78–93). Westport, CT: Greenwood Press.

Matsakis, A. (1997). *Trust after trauma: A guide to relationships for survivors and those who love them.* Oakland, CA: New Harbinger.

McCann, I. L., & Pearlman, L. A. (1990). *Psychological trauma and the adult survivor.* New York: Brunner/Mazel.

McFarlane, A. C., & Girolamo, G. (1996). The nature of traumatic stressors and the epidemiology of posttraumatic reactions. In B. A. van der Kolk, A. C. McFarlane & L. Weisaeth (Eds.), *Traumatic stress: The effects of overwhelming experience on mind, body, and society* (pp. 129–154). New York: Guilford Press.

McFarlane, A. C., & van der Kolk, B. A. (1996). Trauma and its challenge to society. In B. A. van der Kolk, A. C. McFarlane, & L. Weisaeth (Eds.), *Traumatic stress: The effects of overwhelming experience on mind, body, and society* (pp. 24–45). New York: Guilford Press.

Mikulincer, M. (1995). Attachment style and the mental representation of the self, *Journal of Personality and Social Psychology, 69,* 1203–1215.

Mikulincer, M. (1997). Adult attachment style and information processing: Individual differences in curiosity and cognitive closure. *Journal of Personality and Social Psychology, 72,* 1217–1230.

Mikulincer, M. (1998). Attachment working models and the sense of trust: An exploration of interaction goals and affect regulation. *Journal of Personality and Social Psychology, 74,* 1209–1224.

Mikulincer, M., Florian, V., & Weller, A. (1993). Attachment styles, coping strategies, and post-traumatic psychological distress. *Journal of Personality and Social Psychology, 64,* 817–826.

Mikulincer, M., & Nachshon, O. (1991). Attachment styles and patterns of self-disclosure. *Journal of Personality and Social Psychology, 61,* 321–332.

Millikin, J., & Johnson, S. M. (2000). Telling tales: Disquisitions in emotionally focused therapy. *Journal of Family Psychotherapy, 2,* 75–79.

Neimeyer, R. A. (1993). An appraisal of constructivist psychotherapies. *Journal of Consulting and Clinical Psychology, 61,* 221–234.

Nelson, B., & Wampler, K. (2000). Systemic effects of trauma in clinic couples: An exploratory study of secondary trauma resulting from childhood abuse. *Journal of Marital and Family Therapy, 26,* 171–184.

Newman, E., Kaloupek, D. G., & Keane, T. M. (1996). Assessment of posttraumatic stress disorder in clinical and research settings. In B. A. van der Kolk, A. C. McFarlane, & L. Weisaeth (Eds.), *Traumatic stress: The effects of overwhelming experience on mind, body, and society* (pp. 242–275). New York: Guilford Press.

Nichols, M. P. (1987). *The self in the system: Expanding the limits of family therapy.* New York: Brunner/Mazel.

Norris, F. H. (1992). Epidemiology of trauma: Frequency and impact of different potentially traumatic events on different demographic groups. *Journal of Consulting and Clinical Psychology, 60,* 409–418.

Ornish, D. (1998). *Love and survival: Eight pathways to intimacy and health.* New York: Harper Perennial.

Paivio, S., & Nieuwenhuis, J. A. (2001). Efficacy of emotion focused therapy for adult survivors of child abuse: A preliminary study. *Journal of Traumatic Stress, 14,* 109–127.

Paivio, S., & Shimp, L. (1998). Affective change processes in therapy for PTSD stemming from childhood abuse. *Journal of Psychotherapy Integration, 8,* 211–229.

Parker, G., & Hadzi-Pavlovic, D. (1984). Modification of levels of depression in mother-bereaved women by parental and marital relationships. *Psychological Medicine, 14,* 125–135.

Pasch, L. A., & Bradbury, T. N. (1998). Social support, conflict and the development of marital dysfunction. *Journal of Consulting and Clinical Psychology, 66,* 219–230.

Pearlman, L. A., & Saakvitne, K. W. (1995). *Trauma and the therapist.* New York: Norton.

Pennebaker, J. W. (1985). Traumatic experience and psychosomatic disease: Exploring the psychology of behavioral inhibition, obsession and confiding. *Canadian Psychology, 26,* 82–95.

Perry, S., Difade, J., Musngi, G., Frances, A., & Jacobsberg, L. (1992). Predictors of posttraumatic stress disorder after burn injury. *American Journal of Psychiatry, 149,* 931–935.

Plutchik, R. (2000). *Emotions in the practice of psychotherapy.* Washington, DC: APA Press.

Prochaska, J. O., Norcross, J. C., & DiClemente, C. C. (1994). *Changing for good.* New York: William Morrow.

Read, J. (1997). Child abuse and psychosis: A literature review and implications for clinical practice. *Professional Psychology: Research and Practice, 28,* 448–456.

Real, T. (1997). *I don't want to talk about it. Overcoming the secret legacy of male depression.* New York: Fireside Press.

Resnick, H. S., Kilpatrick, D. G., Dansky, B. S., Saunders, B. E., & Best, C. L. (1993). Prevalence of civilian trauma and posttraumatic stress disorder in a representative national sample of women. *Journal of Consulting and Clinical Psychology, 61,* 984–991.

Resnick, P., Jordan, C., Girelli, S., Hutter, C., & Marhoerer-Dvorak, S. (1988). A comparative outcome study of behavioral group therapy for sexual assault victims. *Behavior Therapy, 19,* 385–401.

Riggs, D. S., Byrne, C., Weathers, F., & Litz, B. (1998). The quality of intimate relationships of male Vietnam veterans: Problems associated with posttraumatic stress disorder. *Journal of Traumatic Stress, 11,* 87–101.

Riggs, D. S., Rothbaum, B. O., & Foa, E. B. (1995). A prospective examination of symptoms of post-traumatic stress disorder in victims of non-sexual assault. *Journal of Interpersonal Violence, 2,* 201–214.

Rolland, J. S. (1994). In sickness and in health: The impact of illness on couples' relationships. *Journal of Marital and Family Therapy, 20,* 327–347.

Rolland, J. S. (1999). Parental illness and disability: A family systems framework. *Journal of Family Therapy, 21,* 242–266.

Root, M. P. P. (1992). Reconstructing the impact of trauma on personality. In L. S. Brown & M. Ballou (Eds.), *Personality and psychopathology: Feminist reappraisals* (pp. 229–265). New York: Guilford Press.

Rothbaum, B. O., & Foa, E. B. (1996). Cognitive-behavioral therapy for posttraumatic stress disorder. In B. A. van der Kolk, A. C. McFarlane, & L. Weisaeth (Eds.), *Traumatic stress: The effects of overwhelming experience on mind, body, and society* (pp. 491–509). New York: Guilford Press.

Rothbaum, F., Weisz, J., Pott, M., Miyake, K., & Morelli, G. (2000). Attachment and culture: Security in the United States and Japan. *American Psychologist, 55,* 1093–1104.

Rusbault, C. E., Verette, J., Whitney, G. A., Slovik, L. F., & Lipkus, I. (1991). Accommodation processes in close relationships. *Journal of Personality and Social Psychology, 60,* 53–78.

Russell, D. E. H. (1984). *Sexual exploitation: Rape, child sexual abuse, and workplace harassment.* Newbury Park, CA: Sage.

Rutter, M., & Quinton, D. (1984). Long-term follow-up of women institutionalized in childhood: Factors promoting good functioning in adult life. *British Journal of Developmental Psychology, 2,* 191–204.

Salovey, P., Rothman, A. J., Deitweiler, J. B., & Steward, W. T. (2000). Emotional states and physical health. *American Psychologist, 55,* 110–121.

Saxe, B. J., & Johnson, S. M. (1999). An empirical investigation of group treatment for a clinical population of adult female incest survivors. *Journal of Child Sexual Abuse, 8,* 67–88.

Schmaling, K. B., & Sher, T. G. (1997). Physical health and relationships. In W. K. Halford & H. J. Markman (Eds.), *Clinical handbook of marriage and couples interventions* (pp. 323–345). Chichester, UK: Wiley.

Schmaling, K. B., & Sher, T. G. (Eds.). (2000). *The psychology of couples and illness: Theory, research, and practice.* Washington, DC: American Psychological Association.

Schore, A. N. (1994). *Affect regulation and the organization of self.* Hillsdale, NJ: Erlbaum.

Senchak, M., & Leonard, K. (1992). Attachment styles and marital adjustment among newlywed couples. *Journal of Social and Personal Relationships, 9,* 51–64.

Shalev, A. Y. (1993). Stress versus traumatic stress: From acute homeostatic reactions to chronic psychopathology. In B. A. van der Kolk, A. C. McFarlane, & L. Weisaeth (Eds.), *Traumatic stress: The effects of overwhelming experience on mind, body, and society* (pp 77–101). New York: Guilford Press.

Shaver, P. R., & Clark, C. L. (1994). The psychodynamics of adult romantic attachment. In J. Masling & R. Bornstein (Eds.), *Empirical perspectives on object relations theory* (pp. 105–156). Washington, DC: APA Press.

Shaver, P., Collins, N., & Clarke, C. L. (1996). Attachment styles and internal working models of self and relationship partners. In G. J. O. Fletcher & J. Fitness

(Eds), *Knowledge structures in close relationships: A social psychological approach* (pp. 25–61). Mahwah, NJ: Erlbaum.

Shaver, P., & Hazan, C. (1993). Adult romantic attachment: Theory and evidence. In D. Perlman & W. Jones (Eds.), *Advances in personal relationships* (Vol. 4, pp. 29–70). London: Jessica Kingsley.

Shay, J. (1994). *Achilles in Vietnam: Combat trauma and the undoing of character.* New York: Touchstone Books.

Silver, S. M., & Iacono, C. (1986). Symptom groups and family patterns of Vietnam vets with post-traumatic stress disorder. In C. R. Figley (Ed.), *Trauma and its wake: Vol II. Traumatic stress theory, research and intervention.* New York: Brunner/Mazel.

Simpson, J. A. (1990). The influence of attachment styles on romantic relationships. *Journal of Personality and Social Psychology, 59,* 971–980.

Simpson, J. A., & Rholes, W. S. (1994). Stress and secure base relationships in adulthood. In K. Bartholomew & D. Perlman (Eds.), *Attachment processes in adulthood* (pp. 181–204). London: Jessica Kingsley.

Simpson, J. A., Rholes, W. S., & Nelligan, J. S. (1992). Support seeking and support giving within couples in an anxiety provoking situation: The role of attachment styles. *Journal of Personality and Social Psychology, 62,* 434–446.

Simpson, J. A., Rholes, W. S., & Phillips, D. (1996). Conflict in close relationships: An attachment perspective. *Journal of Personality and Social Psychology, 61,* 61–69.

Sims, A. E. B. (1999). *Working models of attachment: The impact of emotionally focused marital therapy.* Unpublished doctoral thesis, Department of Psychology, University of Ottawa, Ontario, Canada

Solomon, Z., Mikulincer, M., & Habershaim, N. (1990). Life events, coping strategies, social resources and somatic complaints among combat stress reaction casualties. *British Journal of Medical Psychology, 63,* 137–148.

Solomon, Z., Waysman, M., & Mikulincer, M. (1990). Family functioning, perceived social support and combat related psychopathology: The moderating role of loneliness. *Journal of Social and Clinical Psychology, 9,* 456–472.

Spanier, G. (1976). Measuring dyadic adjustment. *Journal of Marriage and Family, 13,* 113–126.

Sperling, M. B., & Berman, W. H. (Eds.). (1994). *Attachment in adults.* New York: Guilford Press.

Sroufe, L. A. (1996). *Emotional development: The organization of emotional life in the early years.* Cambridge, UK: Cambridge University Press.

Stein, M. B., Yehuda, R., Koverola, C. & Hanna, C. (1997). Enhanced dexamethasone suppression of plasma cortisol in adult women traumatized by childhood sexual abuse. *Biological Psychiatry, 42,* 680–686.

Stone, M. H. (1990). *The fate of borderline patients: Successful outcome and psychiatric practice.* New York: Guilford Press.

Sullivan, H. S. (1953). *The interpersonal theory of psychiatry.* New York: Norton.

Suomi, S. J. (1989). The development of affect in rhesus monkeys. In N. Fox & R. Davidson (Eds.), *The psychobiology of affective development* (pp. 119–159). Hillsdale, NJ: Erlbaum.

Tarrier, N., Sommerfield, C., & Pilgrim, H. (1999). Relatives expressed emotion (EE). and PTSD treatment outcome. *Psychological Medicine, 29,* 801–811.

Tronick, E. Z. (1989). Emotion and emotional communication in infants. *American Psychologist, 44,* 112–119.

Turner, S. W., McFarlane, A. C., & van der Kolk, B. A. (1996). The therapeutic environment and new explorations in the treatment of posttraumatic stress disorder. In B. A. van der Kolk, A. C. McFarlane, & L. Weisaeth (Eds.), *Traumatic stress: The effects of overwhelming experience on mind, body, and society* (pp. 537–558). New York: Guilford Press.

Twenge, J. M. (2000). The age of anxiety? Birth cohort change in anxiety and neuroticism, 1952–1993. *Journal of Personality and Social Psychology, 79,* 1007–1021.

Valentine, L., & Feinauer, L. L. (1993). Resilience factors associated with female survivors of childhood sexual abuse. *American Journal of Family Therapy, 21,* 216–224.

van Doorn, C., Kasl, S. V., Berry, L., Jacobs, S., & Prigerson, H. G. (1998). The influence of marital quality and attachment styles on traumatic grief and depressive symptoms. *Journal of Nervous and Mental Disease, 186,* 566–573.

van der Kolk, B. A. (1996). The complexity of adaptation to trauma: Self-regulation, stimulus discrimination, and characterological development. In B. A. van der Kolk, A. C. McFarlane, & L. Weisaeth (Eds.), *Traumatic stress: The effects of overwhelming experience on mind, body, and society* (pp. 182–213). New York: Guilford Press.

van der Kolk, B. A., McFarlane, A. C., & Weisaeth, L. (Eds.). (1996). *Traumatic stress: The effects of overwhelming experience on mind, body, and society.* New York: Guilford Press.

van der Kolk, B. A., Perry, C., & Herman, J. L. (1991). Childhood origins of self-destructive behavior. *American Journal of Psychiatry, 148,* 1665–1671.

van der Kolk, B. A., van der Hart, O., & Marmar, C. R. (1996). Dissociation and information processing in posttraumatic stress disorder. In B. A. van der Kolk, A. C. McFarlane, & L. Weisaeth (Eds.), *Traumatic stress: The effects of overwhelming experience on mind, body, and society* (pp. 303–327). New York: Guilford Press.

Van IJzendoorn, M. H., & Sagi, A. (1999). Cross-cultural patterns of attachment: Universal and contextual dimensions. In J. Cassidy & P. R. Shaver (Eds.), *Handbook of attachment: Theory, research, and clinical implications* (pp. 713–734). New York: Guilford Press.

Videka-Sherman, L. (1982). Coping with the death of a child: A study over time. *American Journal of Orthopsychiatry, 52,* 688–698

Videka-Sherman, L., & Lieberman, M. (1985). Effects of self-help groups and psychotherapy after a child dies. *American Journal of Orthopsychiatry, 55,* 70–82.

von Bertalanffy, L. (1956). General system theory. *General Systems Yearbook, 1,* 1–10.

Waites, E. A. (1993). *Trauma and survival: Post-traumatic and dissociative disorders in women.* New York: Norton.

Walser, R. D., & Hayes, S. C. (1998). Acceptance and trauma survivors: Applied issues and problems. In V. M. Follette, J. I. Ruzek, & F. R. Abueg (Eds.), *Cognitive-behavioral therapies for trauma* (pp. 256–277). New York: Guilford Press.

Walsh, F. (1996). The concept of family resilience: Crisis and challenge. *Family Process, 35,* 261–281.

Waysman, M., Mikulincer, M., Solomon, Z., & Weisenberg, M. (1993). Secondary traumatization among wives of post traumatic combat veterans: A family typology. *Journal of Family Psychology, 7*, 104–119.

Weathers, F. W., Litz, B., Herman, D. S., Huska, J. A., & Keane, T. M. (1993). *The PTSD Checklist: Reliability, validity and diagnostic utility.* Paper presented at the annual meeting of the International Society for Traumatic Stress Studies, San Antonio, TX.

Weiss, D. S., & Marmar, C. R. (1997). The Impact of Events Scale—Revised. In J. P. Wilson & T. M. Keane (Eds.), *Assessing psychological trauma and PTSD* (pp. 399–411). New York: Guilford Press.

Whiffen, V., & Johnson, S. M. (1998). An attachment theory framework for the treatment of childbearing depression. *Clinical Psychology: Science & Practice, 5*, 478–493.

Whisman, M. A. (1999). Marital dissatisfaction and psychiatric disorders: Results from the National Comorbidity Survey. *Journal of Abnormal Psychology, 108*, 701–706.

Wile, D. (1981). *Couples therapy: A non-traditional approach.* New York: Wiley.

Wilson, J. P., & Keane, T. M. (Eds.). (1997). *Assessing psychological trauma and PTSD.* New York: Guilford Press.

Wilson, J. P., & Kurtz, R. R. (1997). Assessing posttraumatic stress disorder in couples and families. In J. P. Wilson & T. M. Keane (Eds.), *Assessing psychological trauma and PTSD* (pp. 349–372). New York: Guilford Press.

Worthington, E. L., & DiBlasio, F. A. (1990). Promoting mutual forgiveness within the fractured relationship. *Psychotherapy, 27*, 219–223.

Wynne, L. C., & Wynne A. R. (1986). The quest for intimacy. *Journal of Marital and Family Therapy, 12*, 383–394.

Zlotnick, C., Zakriski, A. L., Shea, M. T., Costello, E., Begin, A., Pearlstein, T., & Simpson, E. (1996). The long-term sequelae of sexual abuse: Support for a complex posttraumatic stress disorder. *Journal of Traumatic Stress, 9*, 195–205.

Index